Praise for *Stronger Than Before*

'Equally as inspirational as it is practical, and backed up by extensive research, Stronger Than Before is a gift to anyone facing a frightening medical diagnosis. Alison Porter walks you through a healing journey that will leave you feeling like you have the ultimate best friend at your side. Alison herself is the kindest person I know. Read her wisdom and take charge of your healing journey.'

MIRANDA MACPHERSON, AUTHOR OF *THE WAY OF GRACE*

'What a superb book for any woman newly diagnosed with breast cancer and what a perfect title, 'Stronger Than Before'. Alison has done a brilliant job of covering all the ways of tackling breast cancer positively, following in the great footsteps of pioneer Penny Brohn. Penny proved her own theory that 'cancer is negotiable,' living for 21 years with secondary breast cancer, telling us that the key to survival was to find the opportunity in the crisis. Well done, Alison, for shining this bright light for those who will follow you on their self-healing journey.'

DR ROSY DANIEL BSC MBBCH, INTEGRATIVE MEDICINE CONSULTANT

'Beautifully written, deeply moving. A go-to book to reach for first if you find yourself with your world turned upside down after a diagnosis of breast cancer. Alison walks step-by-step with you all the way, signposting your treatment options clearly, and unusually, and in my opinion, vitally, also flags the scientific statistics that may not serve you. Essential reading.'

SARA DAVENPORT, FOUNDER OF BREAST CANCER HAVEN AND AUTHOR OF *REBOOT YOUR HEALTH*

'Can a book about cancer, healing and change be beautiful? I think so. There is so much practical information and wisdom in these thought-filled pages, intertwined with Alison's vulnerability and courage to rise. Her journey toward being her own positive influence is truly inspiring. You will be moved and soothed by this book.'

ROBBI ZECK ND, AUTHOR OF THE BLOSSOMING HEART

'Alison Porter's book, Stronger Than Before, is the book I wish I'd found when I was diagnosed with Stage 3 ER/PR+ breast cancer. Alison and I share a very similar view about cancer: it's not something trying to kill you - it's something communicating that your life is out of balance. Alison shares her own story as well as her thorough research and suggestions to help you make sense of your diagnosis, or that of a loved one, so you can find the eye of calm in the middle of the storm. To eradicate cancer, we must take our lives into our own hands and take responsibility for our own healing. While I wish no one was ever again diagnosed with breast cancer, I plan to give them a copy of this book as it is a resource I desperately could have used during my journey to healing.'

BAETH DAVIS, THE PALM PILOT FOR THE SOUL OF YOUR BUSINESS™, BAETH.COM

'Knowing women who've been through this, I know it takes a great deal of courage to look into the eye of cancer and choose an alternative method to overcome it. This book will lead you with integrity through a range of approaches so that you can decide how to heal, stay well and ultimately become stronger than before. Alison Porter is a brave warrior woman, and her life is a living testament of what is possible.'

KYLE GRAY, BESTSELLING AUTHOR OF LIGHT WARRIOR, RAISE YOUR VIBRATION AND ANGEL PRAYERS

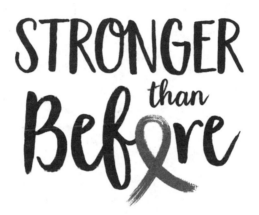

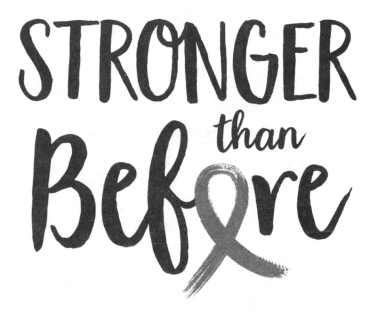

STRONGER
than
Before

Take Charge of Your Healing to
SURVIVE AND THRIVE
with Breast Cancer

ALISON PORTER

HAY HOUSE

Carlsbad, California • New York City
London • Sydney • New Delhi

Published in the United Kingdom by:
Hay House UK Ltd, Astley House, 33 Notting Hill Gate, London W11 3JQ
Tel: +44 (0)20 3675 2450; Fax: +44 (0)20 3675 2451
www.hayhouse.co.uk

Published in the United States of America by:
Hay House Inc., PO Box 5100, Carlsbad, CA 92018-5100
Tel: (1) 760 431 7695 or (800) 654 5126
Fax: (1) 760 431 6948 or (800) 650 5115; www.hayhouse.com

Published in Australia by:
Hay House Australia Ltd, 18/36 Ralph St, Alexandria NSW 2015
Tel: (61) 2 9669 4299; Fax: (61) 2 9669 4144
www.hayhouse.com.au

Published in India by:
Hay House Publishers India, Muskaan Complex, Plot No.3, B-2,
Vasant Kunj, New Delhi 110 070
Tel: (91) 11 4176 1620; Fax: (91) 11 4176 1630
www.hayhouse.co.in

Text © Alison Porter, 2018

The moral rights of the author have been asserted.

The information given in this book should not be treated as a substitute for professional medical advice; always consult a medical practitioner. Any use of information in this book is at the reader's discretion and risk. Neither the author nor the publisher can be held responsible for any loss, claim or damage arising out of the use, or misuse, of the suggestions made, the failure to take medical advice or for any material on third-party websites.

A catalogue record for this book is available from the British Library.

ISBN: 978-1-78817-160-1

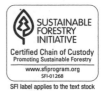

SUSTAINABLE FORESTRY INITIATIVE
Certified Chain of Custody
Promoting Sustainable Forestry
www.sfiprogram.org
SFI-01268

SFI label applies to the text stock

For my mother, who lost her life to metastatic breast cancer as I was learning to save mine.

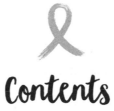

Contents

Part III: Living the Lessons

Introduction

*'When you come out of the storm you
won't be the same person who walked in.
That's what this storm's all about.'*

HARUKI MURAKAMI, *KAFKA ON THE SHORE*

B reast cancer isn't for sissies.

To survive this storm you're going to have to dive deep
to discover every trace of feminine feistiness you can muster.
And if you're up for the challenge, you'll do it your own way.
Your life is at stake – not just the one you had before cancer
swept in like a hurricane, but the one you'll go on to have
when the storm has passed.

The book you're holding in your hands is the one I went
looking for when I first heard those two devastating words
– breast cancer. I wanted a pathway, something to guide me
through this frightening new world of hospital appointments
and fast-paced choices. I read everything I could lay my
hands on – from the most technical medical texts to the latest
in natural anti-cancer diets – but nothing could give me the

bigger picture and help me find my way through the process of treatment and all the painful emotions that came with it.

What I didn't know then was that while every woman's diagnosis and experience of the disease is unique, it is possible to lay out a roadmap that anyone can follow to support them through the process and make the choices that are right for them.

You probably didn't know that there are different types of breast cancer. I didn't. It all seemed like one amorphous disease to me, so I was surprised to discover that there are several different types. And it's a disease that affects one in every eight women. Think of your close circle of friends. If it's not you, then the chances are that you'll be supporting at least one of them through it. And those numbers are rising. While more of us are surviving the disease, more of us are contracting it. We don't just need help in surviving breast cancer, we need help in preventing it too.

The pathway to finding the treatment that's right for you means looking at cancer through a new frame – demystifying it and being open to the possibility that it has a message for you. At first, you'll panic and just want it gone. Then you'll realize that you need to understand the full ramifications of the treatment options you're being given. At this point, your inner feisty feminine will be waking up. During my treatment, I called her the Amazon Queen. She's the part of you who knows how to stand up for yourself, with an intuitive sense of what will work for you – and what won't.

She's an Amazon because, like me, you may have to face the future as a one-breasted woman. And she's a queen because the one overriding quality you need in this process is sovereignty. You will be challenged on a daily basis by people who are certain they know what is in your best interests, but only you can decide what's appropriate for you. You know your body, you know your life, and you know what you need. You'll find your voice and your feisty feminine self-protectiveness, and once it's unleashed it will not be fobbed off with vague explanations. It will ask for proof, and it will not settle until it gets it.

Why do I call it feminine feistiness? Because we need a new model of working with this disease that almost exclusively affects women. All our standard approaches to treatment are masculine and attacking – cutting, poisoning and burning. And the concept of a 'war on cancer' is just as macho. How we think about cancer is through a masculine mindset.

That's not to say those treatments haven't been effective for some. But what if there's a bigger picture and a better way? It's time for a feminine, all-encompassing viewpoint on what is essentially a woman's disease. Instead of battling breast cancer, how about loving your body back into balance? We need a more woman-centric approach that takes into account not just our medical history, but our emotional history too.

Cancer is a malfunction in your body's natural capacity to kill off mutating cells. It isn't something that's attacking you. It's your body failing to recognize mutating cells that it would normally dispose of, creating a disease born of imbalance. Your body's natural defences are failing to do their job. With that understanding, we can begin to look at cancer not as an invader but as a symptom of a body out of balance and in need of support. Then the work begins to look at every aspect of our lives, seeing where balance needs to be restored. To heal ourselves, we're pursuing and creating wellbeing, not fighting a war.

How *Stronger Than Before* can help you

What will you find in the pages that follow? There will be plenty of practical support for the process you've embarked on. Once you've entered the nightmarish theme park that is 'Cancerland', your life has been irrevocably changed. It's a new landscape and you'll need help to navigate it.

I'll guide you through all the key steps in diagnosis and treatment, so you'll understand what's coming, have an opportunity to anticipate the questions you'll need to ask and gain the confidence and tools to navigate a deeply frightening time.

Once you know the lay of the land, we'll delve deeper into all the ways you can support yourself throughout the process. Essentially, this is a book about self-care and taking charge of your healing. How committed you are to caring for yourself will have a huge impact on your recovery and how you move forward into life beyond treatment.

When breast cancer comes along, it feels as if you're suddenly on an unstoppable speeding train. The pace is frenetic. Before you've even had a chance to draw breath, you'll be thrust into making instant decisions on life-threatening issues. There will be a whirlwind of medical appointments and cancer will somehow become your full-time job. You'll be pushed to make rapid choices about surgery, chemotherapy or radiation. Fear will drive you like a demon and your medical team will seem to be in a desperate race to lock down treatment choices immediately. Yet this is your moment to stop, sit back and choose what's right for you. You may be on a speeding train, but *you* get to decide which carriage you travel in.

Breast cancer will take you on a journey that will reveal a lot about you. It will bring things you already knew about yourself – good and bad – into sharp focus, and help you discover strengths that only come to light in adversity. That's why you're reading a book called *Stronger Than Before*. The journey may be frightening, and one that you would never have chosen for yourself, but you'll be transformed by it.

No mud, no lotus. Even the murkiest times in our lives bring dark gifts. A breast cancer diagnosis is fertile ground for a complete reboot of your life. You'll be forced to reexamine your relationship with your body and come to a new accommodation with it. And people will surprise you – in good ways and bad.

Your friendships will change and those you're left with will be the most supportive ones of your life. Where you may have always been the one to help out others – often at your own expense – now you'll need to save your energy for yourself. Breast cancer forces you not only to make choices but also to look at why you're making them. When you're faced with a life-threatening diagnosis, only the big stuff counts.

Stronger Than Before is here to help you find your way through every woman's dark night of the soul. Whether you're the patient, a partner, a friend or family member, you'll find advice here that will comfort you and help you to comfort others. When one of us suffers, we all suffer, and so rarely do we know what to say when faced with the 'c-word' that no-one ever wants to hear.

You may wonder how I found the path in my own encounter with breast cancer. Oddly, it found me. I was forced to look for alternative treatments because I already had a weakened immune system and knew that what I was being offered would completely flatten me. I was as worried about the treatments taking me out as I was about the disease. I had to find a new way. It didn't feel like a choice. It was something I had to do. And the more I researched, the more I realized there had to be another way.

As a coach and a spiritual counsellor, I knew that a diagnosis this shattering would force me to find an inner strength to guide me through – and that it would challenge me to look at anything in my life that I'd brushed under the carpet. Transformation doesn't come for free. But on the other side of it all is a life of much greater meaning and happiness.

That is my wish for you. That your wellness is restored and that your dance with breast cancer brings you a life in full bloom. Our stories may differ, but the path we tread is the same. May this book illuminate your own unique path to healing and help make your journey an easier one.

PART I

WELCOME to CANCERLAND

CHAPTER 1

The Gathering Storm

Understanding breast cancer and finding your feminine feistiness

'I write for those women who do not speak, for those who do not have a voice because they were so terrified, because we are taught to respect fear more than ourselves. We've been taught that silence would save us, but it won't.'

AUDRE LORDE

I found my breast cancer by accident. I'd had a clear mammogram only a couple of months earlier, and cancer was the last thing on my mind. I'd planned a longed-for trip to Mauritius as a reward for a year of unrelenting work, and was looking forward to sunshine, sleep and nothing to do but read.

A couple of days before the flight, as I was sorting out clothes to pack, I reached for something and suddenly realized that my right breast felt solid and quite hard to the touch. I immediately checked the other one and there was a very obvious difference in how it felt.

At an emergency appointment that same day, my doctor thought it was probably a cyst, but she arranged an appointment for me at a breast cancer clinic the next day. There I saw the registrar, who immediately ordered a mammogram, ultrasound and biopsy. He couldn't give a clear diagnosis without the test results, but told me that the ultrasound technician had thought the lump was suspicious.

In possibly the most challenging test of mindfulness I've ever experienced, I had to try to enjoy a fortnight's holiday without letting a potential cancer diagnosis dog my every waking moment. I had to put it out of my mind, because if I returned home and all was well, I'd have wasted my much-needed break worrying. If it went the other way, I needed to be rested to prepare for the onslaught to come. Either way, fretting about cancer wasn't going to help. Of course it wasn't possible to completely forget about it, but I kept an open mind about the likely outcome as best I could.

That began to change as soon as the plane touched down on my way home. I turned on my phone and a text came through, bringing forward the appointment for my test results. When I arrived at the clinic, I was called to see a surgeon, not a registrar. As I walked down the hall to the consulting room, I knew this was not going to be good news.

As the surgeon began to explain what they'd found, my eyes began an involuntary and unstoppable stream of tears. She was very kind and I was quite calm – asking questions and not even feeling as though I were really crying – but the tears just kept coming. No matter how much you think you've got it together, a cancer diagnosis is a body blow and your body is going to react.

Those tears carried on all the way home. Despite my sense of foreboding, I'd gone to my diagnosis appointment on my own and had driven myself there. I then had to drive home, in shock and in tears all the way.

Now that you've entered this life-shattering storm yourself, let's talk about what to expect during diagnosis, and take a look at the different types of breast cancer. Not all cancers are the same, and nor are all diagnoses. You may have caught yours at an early stage, or – like mine – it may be a slow-growing cancer.

All the medical information you'll come across in this chapter and those that follow is the result of my obsession with research. To make it easier for you, I've pulled together information from a number of medical sources and put it into my own words to make it more accessible. Where I've mentioned statistics – or when it's useful to see a study in full – you'll find references, so you can follow those threads if they interest you.

If you want to get a deeper understanding of your particular type of cancer, sites such as www.breastcancercare.org.uk, www.bcna.org.au and www.breastcancer.org are all good starting points. It's only possible for me to give a broad overview here.

Of course, I'm not a doctor and I won't be dispensing medical advice. My aim is to help you to understand what's on offer, support you in deciding what's right for you, and to provide tips and techniques for healing your body, emotions, mind and spirit.

Breast cancer symptoms

First of all, let's take a quick look at the symptoms of breast cancer and see how they differ from the common assumption that we should all be looking for lumps. Perhaps the most shocking aspect of the disease is that you can be going about your life, blissfully unaware of its presence. The signs can be very subtle, and the chances are that you may not feel ill at all. You could experience any or all of the symptoms listed here, or be entirely blindsided by a diagnosis resulting from a breast cancer screening programme like mammography.

The first symptom you may notice could be a change in the appearance of a breast. As I did, you may find a swelling and perhaps a different texture to your breasts. I'd noticed in passing some time before my diagnosis that one breast was larger than the other, but as that's common in many women I didn't really look carefully at the change in breast size. So, here's tip number one – pay attention to any differences between each breast and keep an eye out for changes.

Dimpling in the skin of your breast can be another sign. It might look like the skin of an orange or have an indentation. Pay attention to your nipples too. A discharge from the nipple is a cause for concern, as is a tendency to invert. While many women do have inverted nipples throughout their lives, what you're looking for is something new. Don't be too concerned if your breasts have always been that way.

Any sores, redness or feelings of heat in your breasts should be checked out. In particular, watch out for a rash or what looks like a bruise on your breast, as these are common symptoms of inflammatory breast cancer – a fast-growing type. If you're experiencing any pain in your breast that's unlike what you normally have during your monthly cycle, be sure to investigate that too.

What they don't tell you

Guidelines for when and how often women should be screened for breast cancer with mammography are changing around the world, due to concerns that the risks outweigh the benefits. The Swiss Medical Board now advises against routine mammogram screening, after concluding that there was no evidence to suggest that overall mortality was affected, while emphasizing the harm caused by false positives and the risk of over-diagnosis.[1]

A 25-year follow-up study of the Canadian National Breast Screening Study showed significant rates of over-diagnosis of breast cancer. Twenty-two per cent of screen-detected invasive breast cancers were over-diagnosed, meaning those women were given unnecessary treatment. The same study also found that annual mammography in women aged 40–59 does not reduce mortality from breast cancer.[2]

In addition, mammograms do not necessarily pick up tumours in dense breast tissue – found in around half of women under 50 and a third of women over 50 – and nor does invasive lobular cancer show up clearly, as it usually manifests as a thickening of breast tissue rather than a distinct mass.[3]

Diagnosis

Here in the UK, doctors are obliged to refer any suspicious breast issues to a breast cancer clinic at a local hospital, who will then investigate. At this point it's entirely possible that a lump or change in the breast could be a benign cyst, but it needs to be checked out. This process is similar wherever you are in the world. Your doctor is your first port of call, but you'll very quickly be referred to a specialist team.

At the specialist clinic, you'll be examined by a doctor on the surgical team who may then refer you for further tests. Typically, these include a mammogram, an ultrasound and a needle biopsy to collect a tiny amount of tissue for laboratory testing. Depending on the clinic, these tests could all happen on the same day, but a full diagnosis with lab results will take some time to come through.

What they don't tell you

In a study of 663 breast cancer cases by the John Wayne Cancer Institute in the US published in 2004, those who had needle biopsies before surgery were found to have a 50 per cent greater likelihood of their cancer spreading to the sentinel node – the first lymph node reached by metastasis – than those who went directly to surgery without biopsy.[4]

There are a number of types of biopsy, with varying degrees of invasiveness, ranging from fine needle aspiration to core needle, vacuum-assisted and large core biopsies. Talk to your doctor before you undergo testing, to ensure you're fully aware of the benefits of the procedures and any risks associated with them.

You may only wait a couple of days for the test results, depending on where you're being treated. At your next appointment, a member of the surgical team will talk you through the results and give you a diagnosis. This is your opportunity to discover the type of cancer you have and get an assessment of the stage it is at. You may discuss general approaches to treatment in this appointment, but it's more likely that the next appointment with a surgeon or oncologist will cover this in greater detail.

Diagnosis tips

Take someone with you to your appointment. Do not try to brave this one out. If the news is good, you can go off and celebrate together. If it's not, you'll have someone to lean on, who can listen to what the doctor says, and take you home.

Diagnosis is a shock. You may not fully hear what's being said or recall the details. Having someone with you for diagnosis is one of the greatest acts of self-care you can do for yourself.

To help you understand your particular breast cancer, here's a quick overview of the different types and where they originate in the breast.

Types of breast cancer

Before you begin to panic about symptoms and diagnosis, let's be clear about one thing – breast cancer doesn't necessarily kill you. Only metastatic breast cancer can. It's called metastasis when cancer cells spread to another part of the body, typically the bones, lungs, liver or brain. If your cancer is contained within your breast, your life is not immediately at risk.

According to the Metastatic Breast Cancer Network, only approximately 6–10 per cent of new breast cancer cases are initially diagnosed as metastatic.[5] Even those cases that later become metastatic are estimated to be confined to a range of 20–30 per cent of all cases. Breast cancer is not necessarily a death sentence. Take a deep breath and stay in the here and now. You have time to thoroughly understand your type of breast cancer and its risks before you need to leap into treatment.

Breast cancer can be categorized in two ways, as non-invasive (in situ) or invasive. Non-invasive means it does not yet have the capacity of invasive cancer to spread either within the breast or to another part of the body.

Ductal carcinoma in situ (DCIS)

DCIS occurs where abnormal cells have developed within the milk ducts of the breast and have not spread to the surrounding tissue. It is considered the most common type of non-invasive cancer, but was rarely observed before mammography was common.

There is currently a great deal of debate about over-diagnosis and over-treatment of DCIS, as experts now consider that as few as 20 per cent[6] of cases may eventually progress to invasive cancer, yet all are currently treated as Stage I cancer.

Lobular carcinoma in situ (LCIS)

LCIS differs from DCIS in that it isn't a pre-cancer and cannot itself develop into an invasive cancer, even if it isn't treated. However, it is an indication of a higher-than-average risk of developing invasive breast cancer at a later stage, so follow-up is important. Abnormal cells grow within the lobules, which are the milk-producing glands at the ends of the milk ducts.

Invasive ductal carcinoma (IDC)

IDC is the most common type of breast cancer, accounting for around 80 per cent of cases. Unlike the contained version of DCIS, these abnormal cells have spread beyond their origin in the milk ducts and out into the breast tissue.

Invasive lobular carcinoma (ILC)

ILC is the second most common type of breast cancer. Again, this is a cancer that has spread from its original home in the lobules, and out into the tissue of the breast.

Inflammatory breast cancer (IBC)

IBC is an aggressive form of breast cancer that is thankfully extremely rare. Its onset is usually noticeable through a reddening or rash on the breast rather than a lump. As it's fast-growing and tends to spread rapidly, you should consult with your doctor immediately if you recognize the symptoms. Even so, don't panic. Breast rashes can also be a result of fungal infections developing in the fold under the breast, particularly in warmer weather. Don't scare yourself by jumping to conclusions, but be sure to have any rash investigated.

Within these various types of cancer, you may also test positive or negative for the hormones oestrogen (ER) or progesterone (PR), as well as amplification of the human epidermal growth factor 2 (HER2) gene. If you test positive for these factors, there are medications designed to inhibit their effects.

ER+ and PR+

If your type of cancer is oestrogen (ER+) or progesterone (PR+) positive, your breast cancer cells have receptors that can receive signals from those hormones that could promote their growth. As part of your treatment you may be offered hormone therapy to inhibit their production or block their effect on breast tissue. Around two out of three cases of breast cancer test positive for hormone receptors.

HER2

If your cancer is hormone receptor negative, it may test positive for amplification of the gene HER2, where it makes too many copies of itself, and those copies instruct breast cells to over-create HER2 receptors. This is known as HER2 protein overexpression. Medications designed specifically for HER2+ breast cancers act to block the ability of the cancer cells to receive growth signals.

You may test negative for all three factors, in which case your breast cancer is considered to be triple negative, and will not be treated with either hormone therapy or HER2 medication. More than one in 10 breast cancer cases is triple negative.

Breast cancer stages and grades

When your physician talks to you about your type of breast cancer, they will also talk to you about the stage, which is simply a description of how far it has spread from its original site. The grade your cancer is given is a guide to how quickly it's expected to grow. Let's take a quick look at the stages first.

- **Stage I** cancers are relatively small in size. Either they will not have spread to the lymph nodes or will have reached only the sentinel – or first lymph node – to which cancer is likely to spread.

- **Stage II** cancers will be larger than Stage I and/or will have spread into some of the lymph nodes.

- **Stage III** cancers are large – more than 5cm across – and may either be growing into nearby tissue, such as the skin or the muscle, or have spread into a number of lymph nodes.

- **Stage IV** cancers have metastasized, spreading beyond the breast and the lymph into other parts of the body.

TNM staging

You may also see TNM staging mentioned in your notes. This is a numeric staging system that rates tumour, node and metastasis. It's quite a complex rating system so if this information hasn't been made available to you, feel free to skip this section. It's a bit of a techy read, but if you've been given details of your breast cancer's staging it will help you to understand the size of your tumour and whether it's spread to the nodes, and also show whether or not it has metastasized.

- **TX** means that the size of the tumour can't be assessed.

- **Tis** denotes DCIS, which as we've seen is not an invasive cancer.

- **T1** tumours are 2cm or less in width. Within T1 there are various stages. **T1mi** is 0.1cm across or less. **T1a** is more than 0.1cm but less than 0.5cm. **T1b** is more than 0.5cm but less than 1cm. **T1c** is more than 1cm but less than 2cm.

- **T2** tumours are more than 2cm but no more than 5cm.

- **T3** tumours are larger than 5cm across.

- **T4** has four subsets. **T4a** tumours have spread into the chest wall. **T4b** tumours have spread into the skin. **T4c** tumours have spread into both the chest wall and the skin. **T4d** indicates inflammatory carcinoma or IBC, a faster-growing cancer with red, swollen and painful skin.

- **NX** indicates that the lymph nodes can't be assessed.

- **N0** means there are no cancer cells in nearby nodes.

- **N1** indicates cancer cells in the lymph nodes in the armpit, but they are not attached to the surrounding tissue. **N1** has several subsets indicating the number of lymph nodes affected and whether the cancer cells have reached the lymph nodes behind the breastbone.

- **N2** has two subsets. **N2a** means there are cancer cells in the armpit, attached to each other and to other tissue. **N2b** indicates the presence of cancer cells in the lymph nodes behind the breastbone, but not in the armpit.

- **N3** has three types. **N3a** means cancer cells have reached the lymph nodes below the collarbone. **N3b** denotes cancer cells found in lymph nodes in the armpit and behind the breastbone. **N3c** indicates cancer cells in the lymph nodes above the collarbone.

- **M0** means there's no sign that the cancer has spread. **cM0(i+)** denotes no clinical evidence of metastases, but deposits of microscopically detected cancer cells have been found circulating in blood, bone marrow or non-local lymph nodes.

- **M1** indicates that the cancer has spread to another part of the body.

Breast cancer grades

As well as a stage, your cancer will also be given a grade, which can indicate how quickly it may grow. The grade is determined by how your cancer cells look in comparison with normal cells.

- **Grade 1** cancer cells appear the most similar to normal cells, are slow-growing, and are less likely to spread.

- **Grade 2** cancer cells are faster-growing and look more abnormal.

- **Grade 3** cancer cells appear very different to normal cells and are likely to grow faster than Grade 1 or 2 cells.

Clearly, the earlier stages and grades are easier to treat, but don't despair if you're labelled with a later stage cancer. My tumour was huge. At first it was estimated at 10cm, and then in surgery it was discovered to be 13cm. My breast cancer had also spread to the sentinel node. Three years down the line, I'm still here to tell the tale – and as you'll find out later, I didn't pursue standard treatment.

Even metastatic cancers have increasing survival rates these days. Whatever the stage of your cancer, you must take it seriously, but don't let a number scare you into making treatment decisions before you're fully informed.

The questions you ask at this time are vital. It's important to educate yourself as to what's on offer, and to get a sense of survival rates for your particular type of cancer, but my advice would be to avoid asking for a specific prognosis time frame for yourself. Why? Because however positive you may be, hearing a length of time that you potentially have left to live will worm itself into your brain and that will be very difficult to overcome. Keep it general, and focus on how you're going to overcome this, not how long you have left.

Diagnosis questions

Here are a few questions to ask at your diagnosis appointment, to get the full picture.

- What is my type of cancer and what stage and grade is it?

- Is my cancer slow or fast growing?

- Which treatments are you recommending?

- Why do you recommend those treatments for my type of cancer?

- What are the five-year survival rates for those types of treatment?

- Do you have survival rates beyond five years for those treatments?

- What side effects can I expect with the treatments you recommend?

- Do any of those treatments cause secondary cancers?

- If surgery is recommended, will it be a lumpectomy or mastectomy, and how is that determined?

- Is nipple-conserving surgery possible in my case?

- If chemotherapy is recommended, how much does it contribute to a five-year survival for my type of cancer?

- If radiotherapy is recommended, how much does it contribute to a five-year survival rate for my type of cancer?

- *What is the combined effect of all the suggested treatments for five-year survival?*

- *Is this treatment intended to be curative or palliative?*

- *Would you personally choose this treatment for yourself or a family member?*

Taking charge

We are all under a cultural spell in relation to cancer. We hear the word and we instantly think it's life-threatening, even if our diagnosis is early stage and completely treatable. When you're faced with cancer, you're not just dealing with your own fears. You're dealing with the force of a deeply ingrained cultural belief that cancer means death – and it's terrifying.

Whatever you consciously know about your own situation, subconsciously that cultural belief is weaving its web of fear, scaring you with the ultimate worst-case scenario. That's why one of the biggest factors in healing is to overcome your fear, so you can make the right treatment choices for your body and your life.

Your capacity to survive comes from the earliest choices you make when faced with a breast cancer diagnosis. You can let fear drive your choices or you can choose to take charge of your health and do everything possible for your body, mind and spirit to make sure you survive. It won't be as easy as letting someone else take charge, but it will give you purpose and show you how resilient you can be – even in the face of a potentially life-threatening disease. It's going to be a rough ride, but better one where you're in the driver's seat rather than being a passive participant in the biggest challenge of your life.

Calm & Alert aromatherapy blend

For hospital visits when you need to stay calm and take in new information, try using a blend of lavender and peppermint essential oils. Add a couple of drops of each to a tissue or handkerchief and inhale frequently before your appointment. Lavender will calm you while the peppermint oil will keep you alert. Peppermint is quite strong, so add a couple of drops of lavender first, then one drop at a time of peppermint until you find the right blend for you.

The war on cancer

So why is cancer such a frightening cultural phenomenon? Because it's a war that's been waged in the public psyche for almost half a century, with millions of casualties and little progress.

In 1971, US president Richard Nixon announced a 'War on Cancer', yet nearly 50 years and hundreds of billions of dollars later, we still don't have a cure. The majority of the research arising from that war has been focused on cancer as a genetic disease, even though it's been documented that inherited genetic mutations play a major role in only

5 to 7 per cent of all cancers.[7] For breast cancer, hereditary rates are even lower. According to Cancer Research UK, fewer than 3 per cent of breast cancers are caused by an inherited faulty gene.[8]

Yet as far back as 1923, the German biochemist Otto Warburg found that while normal body cells fed on oxygen, cancer cells fuelled their growth with glucose. This discovery, known as the Warburg Effect, is the basis for the cancer diagnostic Positron Emission Tomography (PET) scans, which show where cells in the body are consuming additional glucose. Warburg's findings were the foundation of the metabolic theory of cancer.

However, after the structure of DNA – the molecule that contains hereditary information for cells – was revealed by James Watson and Francis Crick in 1953, Warburg's theory fell out of fashion. The gene-centred approach to cancer research and treatment has held sway ever since, despite having spectacularly failed to deliver its long-promised cure.

But there has been a resurgence of interest in metabolic theory over the past decade, including support from the father of DNA himself. In 2016, James Watson told the *New York Times* that targeting metabolism is more promising for cancer research than gene-centred approaches. He added that attempting to locate the genes that cause cancer has been 'remarkably unhelpful'.[9]

Alongside this Warburg revival, we've also seen research into how diets heavy in sugar can result in permanently elevated insulin levels, which in turn may instigate the

Warburg Effect and cancer. In the 1980s, Lewis Cantley of Weill Cornell Medical College in the US discovered how insulin influences what happens within a cell, and is now beginning to see evidence that 'it really is insulin itself that's getting the tumour started'.

Cantley believes that the Warburg Effect is the insulin signalling pathway gone awry, saying, 'it's cells behaving as though insulin were telling it to take up glucose all the time and grow'.[10]

A new cancer paradigm

The old genetics-based cancer model would have you believe that nothing you do will make any difference – it's your genes and just bad luck. But the science of genetics itself is changing. The advent of epigenetics has brought the new understanding that gene function isn't fixed. What we do in terms of diet, stress and environmental factors can switch genes on and off and affect our capacity to fight disease.

New developments in immunotherapy are moving beyond the old masculine model of cutting, poisoning and burning it out into a new science of supporting the immune system to do its job in disposing of cancer cells. Psychoneuroimmunology shows us that our emotions have a physiological effect and that our emotional states affect our immune function. All of these new developments are hugely empowering for those of us who want to take charge of our healing. They show that we can have a hand in making ourselves an unsupportive environment for the growth of cancer.

As cancer is a failure of the immune system to function effectively, these innovations all point to the understanding that it is a metabolic disease. In itself, that isn't news. Many scientists and doctors have put forward that same theory in the past, but standard treatment has rolled along without change for decades, and generations of women have suffered the consequences. Now, with new scientific developments supporting this approach, we're at a crossroads. No longer can we be passive passengers in the treatment of our bodies, handing over all the power to the physician to cut it out, poison it or burn it out.

The new cancer paradigm urges us to look at our lifestyle on every level – how we eat, how we sleep, how much exercise we get, the toxins in our environment, how stressed we are and how emotionally resolved we are. All of these factors contribute to how effectively our metabolism functions and how our genes are expressing themselves. We have the power to control our health and affect our outcomes.

Waking up the feisty feminine

Unfortunately, changes in understanding come faster than changes in process. If you truly want to be an advocate for your own health, you're going to come up against resistance from those who are treating you in standard care. What we have been talking about is the leading edge of genetic research and cancer therapy, which generally has not yet filtered down into medical systems based on the old model.

That's why you'll need to develop your feisty feminine presence to find your way through the treatments that are offered to you, and to make the choices that are right for you and your body. When you wake up the fierce feminine, you wake up your intuition too. You'll learn to listen to your body and know instinctively if a treatment fits the path you've chosen.

We'll talk more about how you can use this new paradigm to filter your treatment choices – and how to kick-start your intuition for making the right choices – in more detail in the coming chapters. Here and now, though, know that when you take charge of your healing, you're committing to change. You're signing up for taking the reins and being responsible for your health. No more popping a pill and hoping it gets better. *You* now become the authority on your health and in your life.

With change inevitably comes resistance. Sometimes it's an inner one, where you may fear that you're not doing the right thing or that perhaps you should have just followed the well-trodden path. This is where your feisty feminine lights the way – when you're in integrity with your own beliefs, values and knowledge, the path becomes clear. When you step out of integrity, fear drives your choices.

But mostly the resistance will come from the outside. There will be physicians who will use fear tactics to try to force you down the traditional route, or well-meaning friends and family who don't understand your choices and just want you to do what everybody else does. No matter what anyone else may think about it, this is *your* journey and these are *your* choices to make.

Now is the time to circle the wagons, find the friends and family who can support you unconditionally along the way, and prepare yourself for the biggest lesson you've ever had in self-care. You'll find all the tools you'll need to take care of yourself throughout this process in the chapters that follow. Right now – and for the foreseeable future – your number one priority is going to be taking care of yourself.

CHAPTER 2

The Eye of the Storm

Treatment options and how to support yourself through them

'Fate is how your life unfolds when you let fear determine your choices. A path of destiny reveals itself to you, however, when you confront your fear and make conscious choices.'

CAROLINE MYSS

My Amazon Queen woke up the day a male consultant with no bedside manner told me that his team had met that morning and decided I was going to have chemo before surgery. No discussion, just an imperative delivered from on high.

I'd walked into the room expecting to follow whatever was suggested, but that incredible arrogance tripped off my bolshie Aussie feminist attitude in a flash. Seriously? A bunch of blokes with no knowledge of my medical history had made a life-threatening treatment choice for me with absolutely no consultation?

That moment set me off on the path I would ultimately choose – asking questions, learning as much as I could about what I was facing and learning to trust my inner knowing. In that first appointment, the consultant was surprised – and annoyed – to have me question that decision. I asked for information on why chemo appeared to be the best choice, but he wasn't forthcoming with any answers, fobbing me off as best he could.

What he – and subsequently the oncology team, among others – had failed to take into account was that I had a history of repeated episodes of Epstein-Barr and post-viral syndrome, also known as Chronic Fatigue. My immune system was already suppressed. Having been wiped out by those diseases for years at a time, I had a strong intuition that chemotherapy would absolutely flatten me. At a time when I needed a functioning immune system to help me get well, I couldn't risk the wholesale destruction that chemo can wreak.

And there were other considerations. As a single, self-employed woman, how would I cope financially if chemo had me completely bedridden? And the pre-operative chemo was intended to shrink the tumour, but it was suspected to be 10cm, the size of an orange. How much could that actually shrink? And what difference would that make when it was already a large part of my breast? The stats didn't stack up for me, and I chose to go for surgery without a preparatory round of chemotherapy.

In this chapter we'll take a look at all the options facing you. You'll understand how standard treatment works, get ideas for the types of questions to ask, and consider alternatives. You'll get the whole picture, including the side effects that are rarely mentioned. One-size-fits-all is not an effective response to breast cancer, and there are plenty of science-based alternatives to give you a greater range of options.

Cancer treatment is an inexact science. Delve beneath the surface and you'll discover just how little certainty there is in standard treatment. There isn't even a medical 'cure' for cancer. You're simply considered to be 'in remission' if you survive for five years without a recurrence. Even following standard treatment every step of the way doesn't come with a guarantee. You'll be given general probabilities, but they won't be tailored to your body and the outcome will be uncertain. What heals one does not necessarily work for another, and quality of life is rarely considered as part of the mix.

Understanding standard treatment

The standard treatment approach for breast cancer is a combination of surgery, chemotherapy and radiation. For many, following the standard route is the simplest choice. It isn't easy to challenge what you're offered, and you'll need an inner core of steel if you do. Many medical professionals don't look kindly on those who ask questions, let alone those who are willing to pursue other options.

But the choice is always *yours*. You have the right to ask why a treatment is being offered to you and how effective it is likely to be.

Before you make any decisions on treatment, be sure that you fully understand your type of breast cancer, how aggressive it is and how effective the standard options have proven to be. Remember, you can pick and choose any element of the suggested treatment plan and be given statistics on their efficacy, as well as looking at the combined effect of all the treatments you're offered.

The Greece Test

To take the guesswork out of choosing treatments, the RGCC Onconomics Plus laboratory test – also known as the Greece Test – is a science-based option. It will test the efficacy of a range of chemotherapy drugs and alternative treatments on your individual cancer.

Your circulating cancer cells and stem cells are harvested from a blood sample and tested against a wide panel of drugs and natural substances to see which ones cause the highest rates of cancer cell death.

In the UK you'll need a referral from an affiliated doctor in order to have your blood taken and sent to the RGCC lab for testing. The process is expensive, but it can give you clear evidence to support you in making treatment choices. An additional RGCC test called Oncotrail identifies the concentration of circulating cancer cells for specific malignancies like breast cancer, so it can be used as a benchmark and follow-up test to assess your status during and after treatment.

There is an international network for the RGCC lab, so you can easily find information for your region and instructions on how to get a referral at www.rgcc-group.com.

Standard treatment isn't always a three-pronged process. Chemotherapy may be recommended prior to as well as after surgery, or not at all. Or there may be limited surgery, such as a lumpectomy, combined with radiation therapy. This will depend on the type, stage and aggressiveness of your breast cancer.

First, let's talk through the standard treatment options in more detail, and then we'll cover the alternatives. I'll tell you what my choices were – and why – but this is a deeply personal process. Before you undergo any treatment you must be certain it's the right choice for you. That's why I can give you a roadmap, but not a formula.

Your type of cancer may be very different and your health concerns will also be individual. It's vital that you know the potential side effects and the statistics on the effectiveness of any treatments that are being recommended to you. You need to take charge of your health, research your options and become your own authority in the treatment process. Only when you know your choices back to front should you make a decision. No-one else can do that for you.

You may experience a lot of pressure from your hospital team, questioning your choices and trying to frighten you into following the standard path. They do this because it's the system they work within, and it seems that few of them are open to the wider options. It takes a lot of inner grit to go your own way, but the scariest part of cancer treatment is also the empowering part – it's an inexact science.

Your oncologist can give you an assessment of what may happen to you with standard treatment, but they can't guarantee it. They know the general results of clinical trials, but they cannot predict with certainty the results for you as an individual. Treatment protocols are constantly evolving, and as an informed patient you owe it to yourself to be sure that your choices are the best possible ones for your body and your type of cancer, and the most up-to-date. To survive and thrive, you need to be a kickass advocate for your own health.

Surgery

If surgery is recommended – and remember that it may not be necessary for all diagnoses – then you could be offered a lumpectomy or mastectomy. A lumpectomy removes a section of the breast and is usually the option for smaller tumours. A mastectomy removes the entire breast and tends to be recommended for larger tumours. In my case, with a large tumour, my first surgery was a halfway house between the two – a kind of lumpectomy that was in effect a breast reduction, including repositioning of the nipple.

Even an operation as serious as a mastectomy will likely only require an overnight stay. Some smaller lumpectomies can be day cases, where if you are operated on early in the day you may be able to go home that evening. It all depends on the time of day you go into surgery, any complications and how quickly you recover from the anaesthetic.

As well as a full mastectomy, there's also an option for a nipple-sparing mastectomy, which tends to be offered to those having immediate reconstruction or in preventative mastectomies for those carrying the BRCA gene mutation.

The nipple-sparing mastectomy will only be an option for you if your cancer is early stage and hasn't spread to the nipple or areola. It's done for aesthetic purposes, but you must have reasonable expectations about the result. Your new nipple may look similar, but how much sensation returns after surgery can vary hugely.

What they don't tell you

We've all seen the news stories about women with the BRCA gene mutation having 'preventative' mastectomies – often double ones like Angelina Jolie – to avoid developing breast cancer.

BRCA is the genetic breast cancer bogeyman. It's the one we were all scared of, as it seemed to spell a death sentence. BRC1 and BRC2 are genes that produce tumour suppressor proteins. Some specific inherited mutations to these BRCA genes are associated with an increased risk of breast cancer.[1] But a recent study published in The Lancet found that 'there was no significant difference in overall survival between BRCA-positive and BRCA-negative patients at two years, five years or 10 years.'[2]

Sadly, all those women with the BRCA gene mutation who have been terrified into removing healthy breasts actually have the same survival rates as patients who do not carry it. That's a lot of disfigurement and pain for absolutely no gain.

The removal of your breast is a huge step that should be considered only when you've fully reviewed all other options. Research has shown that survival rates between women with early-stage cancer in a single breast who were treated using lumpectomy and radiation were the same as for women given double mastectomies.[3]

Investigations into the lymph nodes to look for any spreading of your cancer may take place in a separate procedure prior to surgery or on the same day as the surgery itself. Either way, prepare yourself for a battery of scans and tests prior to surgery, as well as a short pre-operative test around a week before admission. That test will assess your fitness to undergo the operation and will include blood tests, a blood pressure assessment and an electrocardiogram (ECG) to check your heart function.

If your lymph nodes are removed during surgery, you'll have the added issue of lymph drainage to deal with post-surgery. The lymph needs to find a new pathway within the body, and until it does, it will pool in the breast area and need to be drained. This may continue for several weeks after surgery, and your hospital will have a seroma clinic where this drainage will take place.

In the long term, you may be at risk of lymphoedema – permanent swelling – and will have to take precautions to avoid this occurring. You'll need to avoid trauma to the affected arm, such as scratches, injections or having blood taken. Any kind of compression, like a blood pressure cuff or tight clothing, is also to be avoided, as are lifting heavy items and excessive heat or cold.

Some risks to consider with surgery are infection, reactions to anaesthesia, excessive bleeding, lymphoedema if lymph nodes are removed and loss of feeling where nerves have been cut.

Surgery tips

- Buy post-surgical bras or use a non-underwired sports bra. After surgery you won't be able to wear an underwired bra.

- For overnight stays, take earplugs and an eye mask with you. Hospitals are noisy and brightly lit, so you may find it hard to sleep.

- Choose a friend to be your designated communicator. They can let everyone else know how you are while you focus on resting.

- Set up a hospital playlist on your phone, so you have uplifting and calming music to listen to as you recover.

- Bring loose clothing for travelling home, including a top or dress that buttons at the front. It can be uncomfortable to lift your arms after surgery, so a cape or wrap is a more comfy choice than a jacket.

- Set up your bedside table at home with bottled water and healthy snacks to nibble on, as you may not want to get up much in the first few days. Stock up on easy-to-prepare food too, like fresh ready meals and soup.

Chemotherapy

If your cancer is at an early stage, you may be offered the Oncotype DX Breast Recurrence Score test to guide your treatment. It's a genomic-based individual risk assessment for early-stage breast cancer that's widely available around the world – and can be provided on the NHS in the UK.

Oncotype DX tests gene expression to give you a score for the risk of locoregional recurrence of cancer cells – on the chest wall or in the lymph nodes – and distant recurrence beyond five years. It also assesses whether hormone therapy alone would be effective or if chemotherapy is recommended. The test is done on a tumour sample removed either by biopsy or surgery.

Chemotherapy may be recommended by your oncologist both before and after surgery. Beforehand, the aim is to shrink the tumour. If that's successful, you may be offered a lumpectomy rather than a mastectomy. You'll usually be offered chemotherapy if your tumour is large or your cancer is grade 3, in the lymph, triple negative or HER2+.

Chemo drugs are cytotoxic, meaning they are toxic to cancer cells. But they are also toxic to healthy cells, accounting for the severe side effects associated with this form of cancer treatment. It's most often given intravenously in your hospital clinic, in cycles that run for around two to three weeks, for a period of approximately three to six months.

Here are some of the common side effects of chemotherapy:

- Hair loss

- Fatigue

- Nausea

- Mouth sores

- Diarrhoea

- Weakening of the heart muscle

- Infertility

- Osteoporosis

- Extremely dry mouth and difficulty swallowing

- Dehydration

- Anaemia

- Increased risk of infection due to low white blood cell count

- Nerve damage

- Neuropathy, with numbness, tingling and pain in fingers and toes

- Skin sensitivity

- Bruising and bleeding due to low platelet count

- 'Chemo brain', which manifests as memory loss, trouble concentrating, mental fogginess and difficulty in doing more than one thing at a time

- Chemotherapy also brings with it an increased risk of secondary cancers, such as leukaemia

Before considering chemotherapy as a treatment option, ask your oncologist for a detailed assessment of its effectiveness for your type of cancer. You should be given a clear indication of how many rounds of chemotherapy would be used, how long treatment is likely to last, how progress will be measured and the survival rates – not just for five years, but also longer term.

Also ask about low-dose chemotherapy, which a recent trial found to be more effective at treating certain types of breast cancer, with less likelihood of recurrence.[4] High-dose chemotherapy can promote a tumour's recurrence in more aggressive forms.[5]

What they don't tell you

A study by the Department of Radiation Oncology at Northern Sydney Cancer Centre, published in Clinical Oncology in 2004, found the overall contribution of cytoxic chemotherapy to the five-year survival rate was only 2.3 per cent in Australia and 2.1 per cent in the USA. It also recommended an urgent and rigorous evaluation of the cost-effectiveness and impact on quality of life of chemotherapy drugs to justify their continued funding and availability.[6]

Radiotherapy

Radiation therapy utilizes high-energy rays to kill breast cancer cells, and is used after surgery to prevent recurrence in the local area. External radiation treatments are generally given at your hospital, five days a week, for a period of around three to five weeks.

The side effects of radiotherapy include the following:

• Fatigue

• Soreness and reddening of the skin

• Lymphoedema

• Hardening or shrinking of breast tissue

• Loss of armpit hair

• Reduced mobility in arms and shoulder

• Skin discolouration

• Radiation pneumonitis, with cough and breathlessness

• Heart problems

• Bone weakness, with increased risk of fractures

Radiotherapy is also associated with an increased risk of secondary cancer, particularly lung cancer[7] and leukaemia.[8]

Radiotherapy also impacts breast reconstruction, with an increased risk of complications and lower satisfaction with the results of implant reconstruction.[9] Radiotherapy can make the skin and muscles of the chest less elastic, so positioning an implant to create symmetry with the unaffected breast can be more difficult to achieve, leading to lower satisfaction with the outcome.

What they don't tell you

A 2012 study by the University of California, Los Angeles (UCLA) Department of Radiation Oncology at UCLA's Jonsson Comprehensive Cancer Center found that despite killing half of all tumour cells during every treatment, radiotherapy transforms other cancer cells into treatment-resistant breast cancer stem cells.

Those induced breast cancer stem cells had a more than 30-fold increase in their ability to form tumours, compared with the non-irradiated breast cancer cells from which they originated. So, while radiation is initially effective at killing cancer cells, it has a secondary effect of promoting malignancy.[10]

Hormone therapy

After surgery and other treatments, if your cancer is ER+, you may be offered tamoxifen, a selective oestrogen receptor modulator, to block oestrogen from feeding breast cancer cell growth. This drug is usually prescribed for premenopausal women for a period of five years, given as a daily tablet. It can induce menopausal symptoms such as hot flushes, mood swings, nausea, vaginal dryness and low libido.

Additionally, tamoxifen significantly increases the risk of developing uterine cancer. In the US, a retrospective review of the Yale-New Haven Hospital Tumour Registry from 1980 to 1990 found that 67 per cent of the tamoxifen group developed endometrioid carcinomas or other carcinomas associated with poor outcomes, versus 24 per cent in the non-treated group.[11]

On recurrence risk, a long-term follow up to the IBIS-I breast cancer prevention trial published in *The Lancet* found that the risk of developing breast cancer between years 0–10 was 6.3 per cent for the placebo group, versus 4.6 per cent in the control group. After 10 years, the risk was 3.8 per cent versus 2.6 per cent.[12] The International Agency for Research on Cancer (IARC), a part of the World Health Organization (WHO), classifies tamoxifen as carcinogenic to humans.

If you're postmenopausal, you'll most likely be prescribed an aromatase inhibitor such as anastrozole, also known by its brand name, Arimidex. It inhibits the enzyme aromatase in order to lower the level of the oestrogen estradiol, and is given as a daily tablet. Its side effects are similar to tamoxifen, including menopausal symptoms such as hot flushes, headaches, nausea, fatigue, insomnia and mood swings, as well as joint pain and stiffness. It can also increase your risk of bone thinning, raised blood pressure and raised cholesterol.

Studies on anastrozole tend to be in relation to tamoxifen, rather than versus a placebo. However, in sequential trials where patients switched to anastrozole after two to three years on tamoxifen, there were fewer recurrences.[13]

Targeted therapy

If your cancer is HER2+, you may be offered Herceptin, a drug that blocks the effects of HER2 and encourages the immune system to attack the cancer cells. It's normally given during a hospital visit, either via infusion, where it's slowly released into your bloodstream through a drip, or by subcutaneous injection.

Side effects include insomnia, loss of appetite, digestive issues, hot flushes, headache, dizziness, muscle pain, blood pressure issues and increased risk of infection due to a lowered white blood cell count. Most significantly, Herceptin brings a risk of serious heart problems, so your heart function will need to be checked regularly throughout treatment.

In a study by the San Raffaele Institute in Milan, Italy, published in *The Lancet* in 2011, a four-year follow up of patients treated with trastuzumab (Herceptin) for one year showed a four-year disease-free survival rate of 78.6 per cent, versus the observation group rate of 72.2 per cent.[14]

Immunotherapy

One of the most recent developments in cancer treatment is immunotherapy, which works by harnessing the power of the body's immune system so it can fight cancer. As a relatively new treatment, it's not widely available in the UK and may be extremely expensive in other countries. If you're interested in pursuing immunotherapy, ask your oncologist for information on the latest clinical trials.

New drug treatments

While we assume that new cancer drugs will only become available when they have been proven to be of demonstrable value, new research published in the *British Medical Journal* in 2017 shows that is far from the truth.

Of the 68 cancer drug indications approved by the European Medicines Agency from 2009 to 2013, only 51 per cent had shown a significant improvement in survival or quality of life, with 49 per cent having uncertain benefits. Of the 23 indications that could be scored with the ESMO-MCBS tool – a standardized scale of clinical benefit – the benefit was judged to be clinically meaningful in less than half – 11/23 or 48 per cent.[15]

Those statistics underscore why it's so vital that you become an informed patient and an activist for your own health. Just because a drug is the latest thing does not necessarily mean that it's effective.

Complementary therapies

Before we take a look at options outside of standard treatment, there are a few things you need to know.

First of all, don't go it alone. Find yourself an integrative medical practitioner who knows the ins and outs of standard treatment as well as alternatives. Do not discount how vital their support will be in helping you to weigh up all the options. While you can quite easily find clinical trials for drug treatments, you'll rarely find them for alternatives, so it can be extremely difficult to compare like for like.

Pharmaceutical companies will fund trials for drugs they can patent, but trials for treatments that cannot be patented won't necessarily receive funding. This is where consulting an integrative doctor will be of tremendous benefit – they can help you to hone in on appropriate treatments and tell you about success stories they have seen with alternative options. Your integrative doctor can also assist you with regular testing, so you can monitor your progress with the treatments you've chosen.

Look for survivors with your type of cancer and see what commonalities they have in their approach. You can join social media groups dedicated to healing breast cancer naturally to discover what others have done, or read blogs and listen to podcasts by complementary practitioners and survivors.

A word of warning though – it can be overwhelming, as there's such a volume of information out there. Be discerning about the groups that you join, as they all have a different approach and some can be very judgemental about those who are doing it differently. Get recommendations from your integrative physician as a starting point, and then begin researching those options. If you cast the net too wide in the beginning, you'll risk drowning in a sea of information, which can be both confusing and disheartening.

If you can afford it, consider the Greece Test (*see page 38*). It will test a panel of alternative options, including natural supplements and immune boosters like Iscador against your circulating cancer cells, to give you a report on the best-performing treatments. Choosing cancer treatments can feel a little like a game of pin the tail on the donkey, and the Greece Test can take some of the guesswork out of it for you.

Whatever your treatment choices may be, the tips and techniques in the upcoming chapters on physical, emotional, mental and soulful healing are key to your recovery. To give your body the best possible chance to heal, you must improve your diet, reduce your toxic load, relieve emotional stress, stay calm and focused, and find meaning in the process of healing. All of these factors will greatly influence your outcome.

Cancer is a systemic disease, so you need to take a whole-body approach, not just pop a pill or hope standard treatment will do the trick on its own. You must be totally committed to your wellbeing in every aspect of your life to beat the odds.

Let's get started with an overview of some of the other treatment options you can consider.

Iscador

This extract of European mistletoe, sold under the brand name Iscador, works by stimulating the immune system to combat cancer. A 2001 German study from the Institute of Preventative Medicine in Heidelberg showed mean survival time in the Iscador groups was roughly 40 per cent longer than in the control groups.[16]

It is produced by Iscador AG in Germany and is most commonly used in Europe. Iscador is available on the NHS in the UK, although it's not automatically available in all regions, so you may have to ask your doctor to request it from your local NHS trust.

Iscador AG produces both consumer and practitioner information packs, if you or your doctor require them. Not all practitioners are familiar with Iscador, so your doctor may require further details before prescribing it. You can contact Iscador AG via www.iscador.com/en, where you can also find details of its availability in countries around the world.

Cannabis oil

Cannabis oil is an extraction of resins from the cannabis flower with two main ingredients: tetrahydrocannabinol (THC) and cannabidiol (CBD). CBD has been shown to inhibit expression of the gene Id1,[17] which is believed to trigger the metastatic spread of cancer cells from the breast to other organs. The American Association for Cancer Research has also found that CBD induces programmed cell death of breast cancer cells,[18] making it a powerful option in cancer treatment.

Cannabis oil is widely available in some countries, but restricted in others. Before purchasing, make sure there is a high concentration of CBD – the active ingredient – in the oil. Look more carefully at composition than price, as a cheaper oil may have a much lower concentration of active ingredients. Be aware that THC is the psychoactive element of marijuana, so it's more restricted in its availability and may be illegal in some countries.

You may also see cannabis oil marketed as hemp extract. Whatever the name, the most important factor is the level of active ingredients. Ensure you have good advice from a reputable practitioner who is used to working with balancing the ratios of THC to CBD according to your individual type of breast cancer.

Hyperthermia

Heat can be used as a cancer treatment, by raising the temperature of the tumour tissue to around 40–44°C/104–111°F[19] to damage and kill cancer cells. Different types of energy can be used to apply heat, such as microwave, radiofrequency and ultrasound. Various methods are used, depending on the size of the tumour and how deeply it is located in the body.

Local hyperthermia will treat a small area, regional hyperthermia focuses on larger areas, and there is also a form of hyperthermia where the whole body is heated via thermal chambers or hot water blankets for the treatment of metastatic cancer. Hyperthermia has also been found to enhance the immune system's anti-tumour response,[20] stimulating it to work more effectively.

Hyperbaric oxygen therapy

A session in a hyperbaric oxygen (HBO) chamber exposes the body to pure oxygen and a higher level of air pressure, delivering a higher concentration of oxygen to the tissues. It can be used to promote wound healing and there's some indication that it could be helpful in breast cancer treatment. However, the studies conducted so far were animal-based rather than human ones.[21]

A mouse-model study also found that HBO therapy combined with the ketogenic diet (*see page 90*) could decrease blood glucose and tumour growth, while offering a 77.9 per cent increase in mean survival time[22] compared to the control group.

High-dose vitamin C

According to the National Cancer Institute in the US, the cytotoxic effect of vitamin C – also known as ascorbic acid – involves a chemical reaction that makes hydrogen peroxide,[23] which may kill cancer cells. Studies have shown that it can selectively kill cancer cells without damaging healthy cells.[24] Vitamin C levels have also been shown to be lower in patients with more advanced breast cancers.[25]

Additionally, in pilot studies, natural products including ascorbic acid have been found to significantly increase the cytotoxic activity of the body's natural killer (NK) cells. A therapeutic dose of vitamin C is usually given intravenously, to bypass the digestive issues it may cause when taken orally.

When researching a private IV vitamin C clinic in your region, make sure to look for a reputable clinic – preferably one specializing in integrative medicine – so they can take into account all of the treatment options you're exploring. Any clinician working with you needs to be clear on how any therapy may affect another form of treatment you're undergoing.

Nutritional therapies

While we'll cover anti-cancer diets in the next chapter, here are a few of the cytoxic nutritional programmes that are widely used. The evidence for these therapies is largely anecdotal, without clinical trials, so do research them thoroughly and discuss them with your integrative practitioner before making the decision to follow them.

The Gerson Therapy

Established by German-born doctor Max Gerson in the 1930s, Gerson Therapy aims to naturally reactivate the body's ability to heal itself.[26] It uses an organic plant-based diet, raw juices, enemas and natural supplements to treat what it considers to be the foundation of most degenerative diseases – toxicity and nutritional deficiency.

Gerson Therapy is a hardcore cleanse, so you must be committed to a complete change of lifestyle. The programme includes drinking fresh raw juice up to 13 times a day, taking plant-based meals and natural supplements, and having up to five coffee enemas per day to assist the liver in eliminating toxins.

There are two licensed Gerson clinics – one in Tijuana, Mexico and the other in Budapest, Hungary. Even after a stay at the clinic, cancer patients are recommended to follow Gerson Therapy for at least two years afterwards. Your suitability for this therapy will be determined by the stage of your cancer and the other treatments you've undertaken. Check the official Gerson Therapy website (www.gerson.org) for more information.

The Breuss Cancer Cure

Another juice-based approach is the treatment developed by Rudolf Breuss, an Austrian naturopath, where a combination of fruits, vegetables and herbs are taken in liquid form for a period of 42 days. It encompasses specific juice recipes for various types of cancer, as well as teas tailored for individual cancers. All the information is available in Breuss's book, *The Breuss Cancer Cure*, although you may find spa hotels offering juicing breaks using this recipe.

The Budwig Protocol

This dietary programme was developed by German biochemist Johanna Budwig. Based on her research into fatty acids, Budwig theorized that deficiencies in specific types of fats allow cancer cells to flourish. The foundation of her anti-cancer diet is a blend of omega-3 rich organic flaxseed oil and cottage cheese intended to address those deficiencies.

The full diet also includes organic fruits and vegetables, fish and shellfish, organic grains, fresh juices and, as you may be delighted to hear, even the occasional glass of champagne. You'll find all the details of the diet in the book *The Budwig Cancer and Coronary Heart Disease Prevention Diet*, and there's a wealth of information about it online too.

Supplements

Vitamin D is now considered a key supplement for prevention and potentially for mitigating the spread of breast cancer.

A deficiency in vitamin D has been associated with tumour progression and metastasis in breast cancer, according to a 2016 study.[27] A small clinical trial of women with early-stage breast cancer showed that higher levels of circulating vitamin D were associated with lower levels of Id1 gene expression in tumours. As we've seen with cannabis oil, Id1 appears to trigger the spread of cancer beyond its original site.

A 2017 study also found that vitamin D supplementation can decrease circulating 27HC – a selective oestrogen receptor modulator (SERM) – in breast cancer, suggesting that it can inhibit ER+ breast cancer growth.[28]

Diindolymethane (DIM)

Diindolymethane (DIM) is produced from indole-3-carbinol (I3C), a compound found in cruciferous vegetables such as cauliflower, broccoli and cabbage. It has been found to be superior to I3C as a chemoprotective compound for breast cancer.[29]

A pilot study also concluded that taking a daily supplement of DIM leads to changes in oestrogen metabolism in postmenopausal women with a history of early-stage breast cancer.[30] This makes it a potential addition to the healing arsenal for those with ER+ breast cancers. I3C is also available as a supplement, and you can discuss using DIM or I3C, or both, with your integrative practitioner.

My treatment choices

After my mastectomy I consulted with my integrative physician, who suggested taking the hormone suppressant anastrozole as a compromise, as I had chosen not to have chemotherapy or radiation. She also recommended an array of vitamins and supplements designed to support my immune system in dealing with cancer. They included vitamin C, vitamin D3, krill oil and a plant-based immune supplement.

Not long afterwards, I decided to take the Greece Test. It indicated only a moderate risk of recurrence, so, with the guidance of another integrative specialist, I started taking the plant-based cytotoxic supplements that were found to be most effective for my cancer, which included salvestrol, genistein and artemisinin. Please do not consider this as guidance for your own supplementation, as the results of your Greece Test are most likely to be different and they may be completely ineffective for you.

Along with treatment and supplementation, I also undertook a complete dietary and lifestyle overhaul, with alkaline food, juicing, yoga, acupuncture, emotional healing, reduced stress, mindfulness and meditation – all with the aim of restoring wellness in my body to give it the best possible chance to combat cancer.

You'll find plenty of guidance and exercises to help you do the same in the chapters that follow. Everything you can do on each and every level – physical, emotional, mental and spiritual – to support your immune system to do its job will give you the edge in overcoming breast cancer.

PART II

SUPERCHARGE Your HEALING

CHAPTER 3

No Mud, No Lotus

Breast cancer as a transformative journey

'A sacred illness is one that educates us and alters us from the inside out, provides experiences and therefore knowledge that we could not possibly achieve in any other way, and aligns us with a life path that is, ultimately, of benefit to ourselves and those around us.'

DEENA METZGER

You're not in Kansas now, Dorothy.

Breast cancer blows in like a wicked wind from the West, shaking everything loose and landing you in a strange new world where you don't even understand the language. It's the stuff of nightmares, yet it focuses the mind like nothing else.

My first instinct was to want everything to return to normal. But as we've learned, that isn't the purpose of a storm. As much as you struggle to hold on to normality, the storm keeps blowing and you have to adapt to a new normal – one that's all about change. This is frightening, but ultimately liberating.

For me it was as though I'd lost a layer of skin. I could no longer bear trivial drama. When you have real drama going on that might just cost you your life, you have no patience for the non-essential.

And it forces you inwards. You need to find the reserves of courage to keep you going, and while you're there, you find out what's really important for you. When you're in search of healing, it doesn't happen only on a physical level with treatment. You have to look at the whole picture – taking into account not just your body, but also your emotions, your mind and your spirit.

One day, not long after diagnosis, I sat quietly and asked the cancer what it was. The answer that popped into my head was 'I am everything you never said.'

When you're going through a crisis, the siren call of normality can be helpful at times. I took great comfort in simple things like a coffee with friends, a fun night out with the girls or a light-hearted movie. It's such a relief to have a day off from cancer, which so often feels like it's taken over everything. And understandably, we all just want to get back to the life we had before breast cancer.

But it's not that simple. A cancer diagnosis irrevocably changes your life, and oddly, that can be a good thing. If ever there was an opportunity to look your life right between the eyes and decide what's important to you, this is it. The platitude 'life's too short' suddenly makes sense. It really *is*.

First of all, you'll try to hang on to as much of your old life – and your body – as possible. Then you'll start to loosen your grip and see a bigger picture and a different kind of life starting to emerge. This is going to be a huge journey of transformation where you learn to let go of trying to control the uncontrollable. Breast cancer isn't just a masterclass in self-care, it's a first-class degree in acceptance – learning to not only be at peace with what's happening to you but also to reflect on what it means for your life going forward. You'll discover new strengths and awaken old ones. Who you really are and what's important to you will become your priorities, as other things – habits, fears and dysfunctional ways of relating – all fall away.

To optimize your healing, you'll need to look at self-defeating behaviours that cause stress in your life and limit your options for self-expression and happiness. Having breast cancer is a huge wake-up call to look at how you nourish yourself and others. It's an opportunity for a complete re-set of compulsive behaviour patterns that you may never have looked at before. It will challenge you to examine your sense of self-worth, as well as your willingness to stand up for yourself and what you believe is right for you.

Breast cancer symbolism

To understand what an illness may mean for us, we can look to the symbolic meaning of that part of the body for inspiration. Breasts are associated with nourishment and nurturing. If we're looking at a dysfunction in the breast, we can ask ourselves these questions.

- *What's my relationship with nourishment? Do I give more to others than myself?*

- *What was my experience of being nurtured as a child? Did I feel safe and cared for? Did my needs matter?*

- *Am I good at nourishing my body? Do I allow myself to feel my emotions? What's my inner*

> *dialogue like – do I speak to myself kindly? Do I make my dreams a priority or do I sacrifice them for others?*
>
> *Breast cancer invites us to find an inner locus of nourishment and self-care. We may have offered all our nurturing energy to others or we may have thrown it all into work. The woman who drives herself to perform in her job without considering her own needs is just as self-abandoning as the one who compulsively cares for others at her own expense.*

The cancer personality

From treating thousands of cancer patients in the US for nearly 30 years, Dr W. Douglas Brodie began to recognize personality traits that were consistently present in cancer-prone patients.[1]

These included being highly conscientious and dutiful, with a tendency to carry other people's burdens and take on extra obligations, and having a deep-seated need to make others happy. Cancer patients also experienced a lack of closeness with one or both parents that resulted in a similar lack of closeness with a spouse or others, and harboured suppressed toxic emotions like anger and resentment. They reacted adversely to stress and had an inability to resolve deep-rooted emotional problems from childhood.

We'll work with emotional issues in much more depth in Chapter 5: Emotional Ease, but for now let's just take a look at the lay of the land. How much do you really know about your own emotional patterns? This quiz will help you to get a feel for your emotional landscape and discover the issues or behaviours that are ripe for release.

~ BREAST CANCER PERSONALITY QUIZ ~

Tick the statements below that resonate with you and they'll give you an idea of where you need to focus first to address a cancer-prone personality.

There are no right or wrong answers and no magic numbers to achieve. Your responses will simply show you where you may be lacking in self-care or have unhelpful emotional patterns that need to be healed.

Nourishment

I tend to take care of others more than myself.	☐
I feel uncomfortable saying no to requests from others.	☐
I always try to fulfil others' expectations of me.	☐
I often feel overburdened at home, at work or in relationships.	☐
I feel guilty when I take time for myself.	☐
I often try to prove myself at work, or over-give in relationships.	☐
I find it hard to receive – compliments, gifts or care from others.	☐

Total: _____

Responsibility

I'm always the one organizing and taking charge of things. ☐

I never miss a deadline or let anyone down. ☐

I work hard and regularly go above and beyond the call
of duty. ☐

I feel personally responsible for team projects at work. ☐

I'm a perfectionist at work or in my home life. ☐

I hold myself to high standards. ☐

I expect more of myself than I do of others. ☐

Total: _____

Obligation

I'm always the first to help out, even if I'm busy. ☐

I rarely cancel a meet-up or evening out, even if I'm ill. ☐

I worry a lot on behalf of others and I'm always trying
to help. ☐

I'm the one everyone calls on for help or advice. ☐

I feel bad about letting anyone down at work or
in relationships. ☐

I'll grin and bear social obligations, even when
I don't want to go. ☐

I'll agree to take on more responsibilities, even if
I'm overburdened. ☐

Total: _____

People pleasing

It's normal for me to be relied upon as other people's 'rock'. ☐

I try to manage other people's moods, jollying them on. ☐

I feel more comfortable keeping the peace than doing
what I want. ☐

I'm sensitive to atmospheres and will try to placate
an aggressor. ☐

I'm more attuned to other people's needs than my own. ☐

I always say yes to a request without thinking, then may
regret it. ☐

It's easier for me to go with the flow than stand up for
what I want. ☐

Total: _____

Relationship closeness

I've had a difficult or sometimes tricky relationship
with my mother. ☐

My relationship with my father has felt distant or difficult. ☐

I wish I felt closer to my partner. ☐

There aren't many people I feel genuinely close to. ☐

I find relationships and intimacy challenging. ☐

My relationships feel like they're missing something. ☐

I don't feel I get a lot of support from my friendships. ☐

Total: _____

Unexpressed emotion

My emotions are quite controlled, and I don't express them easily.　☐

I feel resentful about things that happened long ago.　☐

I'm angry with people in my close circle of family or friends.　☐

Work issues frustrate me and really get me down.　☐

I don't feel safe expressing my emotions.　☐

I'm worried that if I start crying, I'll never stop.　☐

I've never said how I really felt about something important
to me.　☐

Total:　_____

Stress overwhelm

I've had traumatic events in my life where I found it
difficult to cope.　☐

Sometimes I feel helpless to change things or deal
with difficulties.　☐

There are days when it's all too much and I don't know
how to go on.　☐

When I'm stressed, I tend to overeat or drink too much.　☐

Rather than deal with a problem, I keep myself busy
with work.　☐

In stressful times I distract myself with TV, social media
or shopping.　☐

I've had prolonged periods of severe stress in my life.　☐

Total:　_____

Unresolved issues

Emotional issues from the past still bother me. ☐

Even when I try to break patterns, I end up doing
the same thing. ☐

I attract the same kinds of relationships over and over. ☐

I encounter the same issues in every workplace. ☐

I have a lot of fears about life and don't often feel safe. ☐

I struggle with standing up for myself and being more visible. ☐

My relationships always work out the same way. ☐

Total: ___

~

Understanding your quiz responses

Now that you've had a chance to reflect on these statements, let's look at how it all tallies up. Are there some obvious sections where you've ticked more statements? Are your responses generally the same across the board or can you see that they are concentrated in a particular area?

Don't be concerned either way. This is simply information to help you understand the state of your internal emotional environment. All these issues are interlinked, so don't use the quiz as an opportunity to scare yourself – it's simply making it easier to see at a glance where your priorities may lie in beginning to work with them. Even if your responses are spread quite widely, the core work is to begin to focus on self-care.

If you look again at the quiz statements, you'll see how many of them are focused on other people. If you're aligned with many of those statements, much of your energy is going out to others and you'll need to refocus on taking care of yourself. This isn't only a key skill for overcoming cancer personality traits – it will also be the personal powerhouse that will get you through the ordeal of having breast cancer.

If breast cancer had one message for you, it would be that your sense of nurturing went awry. Somewhere along the line, you learned to nurture others and not yourself. Perhaps that was modelled for you by a martyr of a mother who portrayed self-sacrifice as a virtue. Or it could have come from the opposite direction with a narcissistic parent who showed you that your needs would never be important, so you learned to only consider other people's rather than your own.

Whatever the breeding ground for this faulty emotional wiring, the result is the same – instead of nurturing yourself, you'll abandon yourself by prioritizing what other people want or need. This can happen in friendships, with families, in romantic relationships and at work. The same dynamic will be at play, but it will appear in different guises. You could be a leader at work, but you may find yourself overburdened and reluctant to let go of responsibilities, and even taking on more. You could be the one who always does the emotional heavy-lifting in your relationships, carrying the weight of your partner's unexpressed emotional issues as well as your own.

You might be the good daughter who always fulfils her obligations to her family, regardless of her own desires or dreams. You could be the mother that everyone else counts on to help out with their kids, who would never dream of imposing on anyone else. Maybe you're the friend who always gets to be the listening ear, but never has anyone listen to her. Your career might be the one that everyone else felt was right for you, but which you secretly hate. You may be caring for an elderly relative or an ailing parent, while feeling guilty for taking any time out for yourself.

Whichever way this pattern of self-abandonment appears, it's the same issue – self-care is a skill that doesn't come naturally to you, so you need to learn it.

Self-care basics

Self-care is learned in baby steps. It isn't just indulging in bubble baths or pampering sessions at the spa. It's a daily commitment to small choices that affirm who you are and what you need. If you have a long history of denying your desires, you may not even know what they are.

Think of learning self-care as an adventure. You'll be exploring your deepest self to discover what you value, what you want out of life and what you yearn to express creatively. You'll be taking a deep dive down into the mud, so that ultimately you can blossom like a lotus flower – grounded in the murky depths of your humanness, but flowering with your true purpose. With self-care, you'll find the solid ground within you to bloom as you were intended, with clarity of vision, a powerful life force and a strong sense of purpose.

Here are some of the principles you need to keep in mind to be sure that you're practising self-care.

Pause before you respond

If your ingrained instinct is to always say yes to whatever's asked of you, learn to take a moment before you respond. Try saying 'Let me get back to you on that' or 'I need to check my diary.' Use any quick holding statement that allows you to feel comfortable to take a break before responding.

Then, when you've had a chance to feel into whether you'd like to do it or not, you can respond from a position of authentic choice, not a knee-jerk reaction. Every self-affirming choice that you make adds a deposit into the self-care bank, helping you to build a strong sense of what's right for you and what's not.

No choice is too small. If someone offers you coffee, say 'Let me think for a minute' and decide if you'd prefer tea or a cold drink. Even tiny decisions like this will exercise your self-care muscle and put you in touch with how you really feel. When you're going through treatment or recovering from it, you need to be careful not to overextend yourself, so this practice will help you to avoid overcommitting yourself.

Get comfortable with setting boundaries

Do you have friends who always make demands on you? Work colleagues who push and push until you agree? Family who undermine your good intentions until it's easier for you to do what they prefer? Now is the time to learn how to set boundaries. Good fences make good neighbours. When everyone knows what to expect, it's easier all round, with no room for misunderstandings.

If overwork is a problem for you, set a time that you'll always leave the office, regardless of how busy you are. If you have a hectic family life and no-one's helping, make it clear that you won't clean up after them anymore. If a friend always moans for hours on the phone, tell them you're heading out in 10 minutes, and make sure you draw the conversation to a close when the time is up.

Boundaries make it clear for everyone about what you're willing to do and what you're not. Those fences don't just keep people out – they preserve the space that you need to rest, to be yourself, to reflect and to heal.

Let others be responsible for themselves

No matter how much you love them and want to help them, the people around you at home and at work will continue to repeat their patterns and make their own mistakes. Let them. Worrying about them incessantly doesn't help you or them, and you aren't responsible for their lives. You can care about someone and offer advice or assistance if they're open to it, but after that you need to step away and focus on your own life.

Your energy is needed for your own healing, so you must reverse the pattern of always focusing outwards on others. Think of your energy as a finite resource. You can't keep giving from an empty well, and you can't heal yourself if you're depleted. Having breast cancer is a surprisingly emotional experience. You'll find yourself more drained by it than you might have expected, so remember that energy is the currency of healing and keep your reserves for yourself.

Learn to let go

It's not just people you need to leave to their own devices, it's everything you've felt overly responsible for too. If you're the one everyone counts on to organize celebrations or plan trips, then someone else is going to have to step up to the plate. If you think it absolutely needs to be done by you, you're probably wrong. Somebody else can pick up the slack. Maybe you're always the one who takes on a particular responsibility at work. Or perhaps you're the one in your group of friends that everyone relies on to make bookings for nights out. Whatever responsibilities you've taken on out of a sense of obligation, let them go.

A period of healing is when you need to be gentle with yourself, and you need lots of time and space for rest and recuperation. A diary full of obligations will weigh you down. You can use your healing time as a rare opportunity to start rebuilding your life from the ground up, only taking on what you're genuinely happy to do. It's a new beginning and a chance to source your life from joy, not obligation.

Let yourself be supported

The pattern of not allowing support in your life can be tough to break. If you're the independent type or the one who is always taking care of others, you probably won't be comfortable with being supported. You're used to being the one who gives, not the one who receives. But this is just a pattern of behaviour, and patterns can be broken. It's going to feel awkward and a little uncomfortable for you at first because it's a new way of being, but you need to persevere.

On a practical level, recovering from treatment can be a lengthy process and you may require a lot of physical help. It can feel a little strange to ask for assistance, but remember that others enjoy being able to help you as much as you've taken pleasure in helping them.

There are so many small things you can do to make your life easier too – order groceries online so you don't have to drag yourself around the supermarket when you're tired, stock up on healthy ready meals for low-energy days, hire a cleaner and ask for help with taking children to school or walking the dog.

Keep asking yourself, *How can I make this easier?* and *Who can help?* The key point here is not to just wait for people to offer, but to learn to ask for help when you need it. In asking for what you need, you're sending yourself a clear message that your needs are important and you're willing to put yourself first.

Get connected

We've talked a lot about distancing yourself from draining people to make space for your healing, but making sure you nurture supportive friendships and close relationships with your partner and family is just as important. Learning to discriminate between those who are focused only on their own needs and those who treat you well is a vital skill in recovery. Good self-care means healthy relationships with people you feel close to, and that you can be open and honest with when the going gets tough. Your spirits will stay high when you can share the load.

This isn't the time to try to manage other people's emotions. Choose to spend your time with the people who are supportive on all levels, not only with their words but also with their time and energy. Your personal relationships can deepen when you go through this together. A loving circle of friends and family can ease the isolation you can feel when you're going through a traumatic time. They won't necessarily understand fully, because breast cancer raises a lot of emotional issues about femininity that only those who've experienced it will really get, but they can stand by your side and you can lean on their strength when you're having a wobble.

Learn to nourish yourself

If you have a habit of dialling down your needs so low that you don't even recognize them anymore, your healing time is a chance to reconnect with yourself, without all the distractions of day-to-day life.

Take moments throughout the day to check in with how you're feeling. Notice if you've been pushing yourself. Pay attention to when you're tired or hungry, and don't try to push through. Learn to live at a gentler pace that gives you the space to stay in touch with what you need. Notice how you feel after spending time with people. Spend more time with those who uplift you and avoid those who don't.

Feel into what your body needs, and nourish it with enticing, fresh food. Surround yourself with the things that bring you joy and make you smile. Be aware of your own comfort.

Treat yourself gently. Spend time in nature and indulge your senses. Take time out to read a novel, watch movies or just give yourself empty space to potter and muse. No more running on empty – notice what fills you up and give it to yourself without guilt.

Set aside self-attack

That voice in your head that tells you you're not doing it right, could be doing it better or should have taken better care of yourself is not you. It's an internalized replay of the critical voices of others that you've been regurgitating for so long that you've forgotten it's not you at all.

During your healing time, more than ever, it's so important to be self-accepting, not self-attacking. When that voice starts up, recognize it for what it is – some mouldy old criticism long past its sell-by date. You don't need to fight it. You can give it a name – preferably one that amuses you – then thank it for sharing, and move on.

If the 'what ifs' start playing in your head, accusing you of not doing enough to take care of your health and making this illness your fault, acknowledge those thoughts, but don't give them power. Say to yourself, *I did the best I knew before, and now I'm taking charge of my healing.* No-one really knows all the reasons why cancer develops, so let yourself off the hook for not having done better in the past. As you learn and grow in wellness, you may have thoughts of regret, but let them pass. What's important is that you're in charge of your healing and your life now.

Self-care can become the foundation of your life. Every time you shift out of your automatic responses and into self-compassionate action, you're strengthening that foundation. It takes time, and you'll slip often – particularly if you're tired. We all know how our resolve slips when we have little energy, and all our good intentions go out the window. Even when that happens, it's another opportunity for self-care. Choose to be kind to yourself.

Learn to be compassionate with your body, your thoughts and your emotions. When it's all too much, rest. When it's too stressful, take a break and indulge in something that makes you feel nourished. When your emotions are running high, accept them and let them flow. However you feel, be OK with it. You're healing. It's a process, and the only way out is through.

On the other side of all of this, you can have a greater sense of empowerment and purpose. You'll know who you truly are and you'll surprise yourself with what you can endure with grace. That doesn't make it a pleasant process, but it's a transformative one that can leave you stronger than before.

Now that you have a rough sense of what this illness is trying to tell you, and how to take care of yourself and your needs, let's move on to the steps you can take on a physical level to heal your body.

CHAPTER 4

Embodiment

Befriending your body and helping it to heal

'And suddenly, lying in bed, I became aware of every inch of my body and I apologised to it, quietly. I apologised for being so ungrateful for so long.'

FRANCESCA MARTÍNEZ

My relationship with my body was combative long before breast cancer. Growing up in outdoorsy Australia, surrounded by surfie blondes, I was a fish out of water as a bookish redhead. While my friends could hang out at the beach all day, I could burn to a crisp in an hour or two.

My teenage breasts were at first all-too-flat, then suddenly arrived with a vengeance when the ideal body shape was still Twiggy-esque. My mother had her own battles with body image and was enormously critical if I put on any weight. By the end of my teens I'd diced with eating disorders and found myself disconnected from my body, living in my head.

Throughout the years, like most women, I punished my body with every diet going. I didn't know how to nurture it, but I knew how to batter it into submission. Sporadic gym memberships came and went, and I would spend money on whatever went on the outside – clothes, skincare, haircare – but still there was no inner connection to my physical being.

I was pursuing spirituality and mindfulness from my earliest teenage years, but that was an escape from the body, not an entry point into it. Several episodes of chronic illness – Epstein-Barr, Chronic Fatigue Syndrome and Fibromyalgia – debilitated my body for years. I looked for solutions wherever I could find them and slowly got well, but still my body and I were at war. Paradoxically, it took breast cancer and the loss of my breast to make peace with it.

You've already learned the essential truth of this disease – breast cancer is a crash-course in self-care. If you've ever struggled with the motivation to treat yourself well, you've just found it. Nourish and nurture are now your mission. Your life depends on it.

> *'When a flower doesn't bloom,*
> *you fix the environment in which*
> *it grows, not the flower.'*
>
> ALEXANDER DEN HEIJER

Nutrition

The first act of nourishment for a body under siege is good nutrition. Cleaning up the way you eat is your top priority. Your body needs all the support it can get to fight this disease, so the first things to go are those that stress it and make its job more difficult. Remember, cancer is a systemic disease. Something's rotten in the state of Denmark. Your body's defences aren't functioning normally, so you have to do everything in your power to support your immune system to perform its job effectively.

Think of your body as the ground in which health blooms. Like a fine wine that can only be produced from an optimal *terroir* – the soil with the ideal nutrients and a microclimate that supports growth – so your body must become the ideal environment for your wellbeing to blossom. When you bring your body back into balance, it can resume its role in destroying cancer cells as they arise. Immunotherapy – currently the leading-edge cancer treatment – uses this premise to empower the immune system to combat cancer cells.

Your immune system

Usually the only time we think about our immune system is when we're sick. We know we need it to fight off illness, but rarely do we think about where it resides in the body.

A 1999 scientific paper published in the American Journal of Physiology by doctors from the University of Melbourne found that 'the gut immune system has 70–80 per cent of the body's immune cells.'[1] If your gut health is poor, your immune system function will automatically be impaired. Keeping yourself well nourished with foods that don't stress the gut is vital in combatting cancer.

If you're sceptical about how much diet and lifestyle can affect breast cancer rates, a 1993 study on migration patterns and breast cancer risk for Asian-American women is an eye-opener. The rates of breast cancer in the US have historically been four to seven times higher than in Asian countries like China, Japan and the Philippines, yet when those women migrate to the US their risk grows over generations. Asian-American women born in the US have a breast cancer risk 60 per cent higher than those born in the East, leading the study to conclude that exposure to a Western lifestyle had a substantial impact.[2]

The alkaline diet

One of the leading anti-cancer approaches to nutrition is the alkaline diet. During digestion, alkaline foods such as fresh fruits, vegetables and nuts break down into short-chain fatty acids containing prebiotics that nourish the good bacteria in the gut. This helps to reduce inflammation in the body, which can contribute to cancer. Additionally, as the microenvironment of tumours has been found to be generally more acidic than normal tissue, it's believed that acid pH may influence the outcome of tumour therapy.[3]

On an alkaline diet, you'll be consuming foods high on the pH scale, with 0 being the most acidic and 14 being the most alkaline. Our modern diet is heavily skewed towards the acidic end of the scale – packed with acidic animal proteins, dairy, grains and sugars – so to redress the balance an alkaline diet is largely plant-based. Apart from its general health and potential cancer benefits, the alkaline diet has been found to increase intracellular magnesium. Available magnesium is required to activate vitamin D,[4] which as we've seen, can be breast-cancer protective.

The general principles of the alkaline diet are to eat mostly fresh fruits and vegetables, stick to whole grains, avoid processed foods, and limit consumption of meat, dairy, sugar and alcohol. We'll be talking about toxic load later, but take it as read that organic food will always be the cleaner, better choice. For recipes and inspiration on how to live well on a plant-based diet, take a look at Kris Carr's book *Crazy Sexy Kitchen: 150 Plant-Empowered Recipes to Ignite a Mouthwatering Revolution*.

Eating clean on a budget

The US-based Environmental Working Group publishes annual lists of fruits and vegetables rated for levels of pesticide residues. Their Dirty Dozen highlights those foods where it's a priority to buy organic because they have high concentrations of pesticides, while the Clean Fifteen lists foods with lower levels of pesticides, so it's less important to pay a premium for organic produce.

At the time of writing, the Dirty Dozen[5] features strawberries, spinach, nectarines, apples, peaches, pears, cherries, grapes, celery, tomatoes, sweet peppers and potatoes. The current Clean Fifteen[6] lists sweet corn, avocados, pineapples, cabbage, onions, frozen peas, papaya, asparagus, mango, aubergine, honeydew melon, kiwi, cantaloupe, cauliflower and grapefruit.

The ketogenic diet

Another upcoming contender for the top cancer-fighting nutritional approach is the ketogenic diet, where a low consumption of carbohydrates puts the body into ketosis, allowing it to burn ketones for energy rather than relying on sugar or carbs. This taps into a key characteristic of cancer cells – they have 10 times more insulin receptors than normal cells, which allows them to feed on glucose at a high rate. Carbohydrates break down into glucose, so by removing them from your diet, you're depriving cancer cells of their energy supply.

The ketogenic diet is currently enjoying a wave of popularity, but as it's in the early stages of adoption, there isn't a great deal of evidence for how beneficial it is for cancer. To be clear, no diet has the absolute seal of approval as an anti-cancer approach, but you'll find many survivors who have gone on to live far beyond their original prognosis after adopting a cleaner, more alkaline diet. It will take some time for similar success stories to filter through for the ketogenic diet.

A cancer-protective style of ketogenic diet has restrictions around carbohydrates and the types of proteins and fats that should be eaten. Earlier versions of ketogenic diets were heavily weighted towards meat and dairy consumption, but a low-fat diet has been found to show a near 30 per cent reduction in the production of estradiol,[7] the oestrogen that brings an increased risk of breast cancer.

Let's not throw the baby out with the bathwater – there are good fats and bad fats, and that understanding lies at the heart of Dr Joseph Mercola's book *Fat For Fuel: A Revolutionary Diet To Combat Cancer, Boost Brain Power and Increase Your Energy*, which is a key resource for an anti-cancer ketogenic diet. It focuses on eating minimal carbohydrates, moderate protein and high levels of healthy fats. According to Dr Dominic D'Agostino of the University of South Florida College of Medicine in the US, to be truly cancer-protective, a ketogenic diet must not only restrict carbs but also calories and protein in order to starve cancer cells of their fuel.[8]

Intermittent fasting

Another recent frontrunner as a cancer-protective diet option is intermittent fasting. There are a number of approaches to this – from a simple restricted window for eating of six to eight hours daily, leaving a period of 16–18 hours a day of fasting, to the 5:2 diet and alternate-day fasting.

In the restricted eating window approach, you'll have your last meal as early as possible in the evening and break your fast as late as you can in the daytime, so that your meals fall within a short range of time. In the 5:2 diet, calories are restricted to 500 for two days per week, with five days of normal eating.

For alternate-day fasting, you would switch between a day of normal eating and a day where calories are restricted to 500. Intermittent fasting is believed to be anti-inflammatory and immune supportive, and a 2015 study found that prolonged nightly fasting could be a simple strategy for reducing the risk of breast cancer recurrence.[9]

One caveat here – the normal diet in intermittent fasting must take into account the dietary restrictions that are so important for those with cancer, such as no sugar or dairy, little or no meat and largely plant-based and unprocessed foods.

Forbidden foods

Whichever dietary approach you decide to follow, there are some foods you simply have to kiss goodbye to when you have cancer. If you do nothing else, then at least radically reduce your consumption of sugar. As mentioned earlier, the Warburg Effect found that cancer cells do not feed on oxygen like healthy cells, but on the fermentation of sugar. If you want to starve your cancer cells, your sweet tooth is going to have to take a back seat.

When we're talking sugar, we're not just considering the processed version. There's a lot of debate about whether natural sugars should also be avoided, so it's probably best to opt for fruits and vegetables with lower levels of sugar where possible. Each diet will have different guidelines on the consumption of fruits and vegetables, so your first priority will be to adhere to the protocol you have chosen.

Dairy and meat should be eliminated or at least severely restricted. A 2017 study compared the Western diet (high in fatty and sugary products as well as red and processed meat), a Prudent diet (high in low-fat dairy, vegetables, fruits, whole grains and juices) and a Mediterranean diet (high in fish, vegetables, legumes, boiled potatoes, fruits, olives, and vegetable oils, with a low intake of juices). The results showed that the Western dietary pattern seemed to increase breast cancer risk, the Prudent diet showed no effect, and the Mediterranean diet seemed to be protective.[10]

Alcohol is another one that needs a time-out on the naughty step. The 2017 World Cancer Research Fund International/ American Institute for Cancer Research Continuous Update Project Report: Diet, Nutrition, Physical Activity and Breast Cancer 2017 found it to be a probable cause of premenopausal breast cancer and a convincing cause of postmenopausal cancer.[11] It's time to get inventive with the mocktails, or simply save that glass of champagne for special moments only. While you're in the process of healing, it's better to avoid or severely limit any food or drink that has been shown to promote breast cancer.

Healing foods

Before it all feels like doom and gloom on the food front, let's focus on the foods that can supercharge your body's ability to heal from cancer. It's as important to know how to maximize your cancer-fighting nutrition as it is to know what not to eat.

Leafy green vegetables such as kale, spinach and watercress are brimming with antioxidants, and cruciferous vegetables such as cabbage, cauliflower and broccoli contain known cancer-preventive phytochemicals. Top of the pops on the antioxidant list are berries, particularly blueberries. Eat the rainbow of vegetables like beets, carrots and sweet potatoes, also known for their high levels of antioxidants.

Spice your food with turmeric, as its active ingredient, curcumin, has been shown to help in the fight against breast cancer. And try drinking green tea, as EGCG, one of its major catechins, or natural antioxidants, has been found to suppress tumour growth in breast cancer.[12]

Food feedback

Make your meals a little more mindful by doing a quick check-in when you eat. If there's a food you think may be problematic, just stop for a few seconds before eating it, take a couple of deep breaths and notice how your body feels. Pay attention to the sensations in your stomach and also notice how energetic you feel. After eating, do the same, and then check in again after about an hour or so. This will help you identify foods that your body finds more difficult to digest. You can then decide whether to simply cut down on them, do an exclusion diet or take an allergy test.

Juicing

When you're unwell and trying to build your immune system, fuelling yourself with large amounts of high-quality nutrients is vital to your recovery. Juicing makes it easy to radically increase your intake of vegetables and fruits.

You can use a traditional juicer, which is ideal for combining root vegetables such as beetroot or carrots with high-water content vegetables such as celery and fruits like apple. Or you can use a high-powered blender to combine green vegetables such as kale with fruits such as papaya or mango, adding water to the mix to turn the flesh into a juice. Try adding a teaspoon of a super-green powder that includes phytonutrients like spirulina, chlorella or wheatgrass to supercharge the nutritional value of your juice and add to the flavour too.

My favourite juice combinations are carrot, apple and ginger or beetroot, celery and ginger, as well as kale and pineapple as a green juice. I also tend to start the day with a blueberry and matcha green tea smoothie made using coconut milk, flaxseed and herbal tinctures like echinacea and milk thistle. Those are my personal choices, but make sure your recipes follow the guidelines of your chosen diet. Again, organic fruits and vegetables are always a better choice, or you could find yourself ingesting a high level of pesticides when you're trying to reduce your body's toxic load.

A word on fruit and vegetable sugars – as we talked about earlier, there are various schools of thought on the risks related to the natural sugars in food. You'll need to weigh that up with whichever dietary approach you're using, and be consistent with those principles.

Digestive supplements

With 70–80 per cent of your body's immune system located in your gut, good digestion needs to be optimized. That means limiting foods that your body has difficulty metabolizing and using supplements to support your digestive process. You can look into allergy and intolerance testing for problematic foods, or use an exclusion diet to assess your body's sensitivities.

You could try using digestive enzymes to support the digestive process, as well as probiotics and prebiotics. Probiotics introduce good bacteria into the gut, while prebiotics nurture the bacteria that are already there. Understanding the influence of the gut microbiome – the vast array of organisms that live in our gut – is a growing area of cancer research. We've seen research on how the gut microbiome can affect mood as well as autoimmune disorders, and the next stage in creating a truly personalized cancer treatment is understanding how the microbiome may influence the development of disease and what role it might play in treatment.

For example, a 2017 study discovered that the breast tissue of healthy women contained more of the Methylobacterium species of bacteria than did the tissue of women with breast cancer.[13] While we're waiting for further developments in this area of research, we can support our immune system via supplementation and by reducing our exposure to the things that impair its function.

Toxic load

In modern life our exposure to known carcinogens – the substances identified as causing cancer – is rapidly growing. In each decade between 1980 and 2010 around 25 new agents were newly classified as carcinogenic to humans by the International Agency For Research On Cancer (IARC). Its latest review lists more than 100 carcinogenic agents, with a number of others considered probably or possibly carcinogenic.[14]

Another peer-reviewed study undertaken by the Silent Spring Institute – which specializes in researching the environment and women's health – has identified the highest priority toxic chemicals that women should reduce their exposure to for breast cancer prevention.[15] They include chemicals in petrol, diesel and other vehicle exhaust, flame retardants, stain-resistant textiles, paint removers and disinfection byproducts in drinking water.

Endocrine disruptors, also known as hormone disruptors, are also recognized as contributing to breast cancer risk.[16] Polycyclic Aromatic Hydrocarbons (PAHs) are types of chemicals formed during the combustion of substances like coal, wood and petrol, as well as in foods such as well-done meat.

Bisphenol A (BPA) is found in plastic bottles and the epoxy resins that line cans of food. Organochloride pesticides are insecticides and herbicides that are widely used in agriculture, affecting our foods. Phthalates are plasticizers that leach easily and can be found in toys, as well as in foods like high-fat dairy products or cooking oils, and cosmetics.

And the list goes on. The chemicals in our environment, the ones we put on our bodies and the ones we don't even realize are in our food are affecting the function of our bodies and promoting tumour development.

Reducing your toxic load

Knowing that cancer is a multifactorial disease caused by an immune system that's out of whack, we must do whatever we can to reduce our toxic load so our bodies can return to their natural, healthy functioning. This means a major review on every level to create a non-toxic environment – what we eat, the water we drink, the cosmetics and body lotions we apply, the cleaning products we use, the air quality in our homes and the chemicals in our furniture.

For food, think organic and non-processed, and avoid canned items. Make sure your drinking bottles are BPA free or use glass or stainless steel ones. Be careful with non-stick cookware too, as it can leach toxic chemicals if the surface coating becomes scratched. Use glass food storage wherever possible, rather than plastic.

Check out the toxicity of your cosmetics and all the lotions and potions you're using on your body. Think Dirty® is a phone app that will give you a toxicity rating for leading brands of cosmetics, helping you to make better choices when you're shopping for make-up and skincare. The Environmental Working Group's online Skin Deep® database[17] also rates over 73,000 products for their toxicity.

Or you can take the worry out of decision-making by opting only for organic brands. Don't be fooled by the word 'natural' on product packaging. It's not regulated and means very little. Find an independent body – like the Soil Association in the UK – and buy products they have certified, or confine your purchases to companies with strong reputations for pure, natural products. Be aware that smaller cosmetics companies are often taken over by large conglomerates, so the reputation you may have relied on can change under new ownership. Be an active and aware consumer, especially for products you're using on your skin.

When we're talking clean water, we're not just considering the source, but also how it's packaged. Rather than purchase clean water in potentially toxic plastic bottles, try investing in a high-quality home water filter. The better ones will filter out a large number of contaminants and create water with a more alkaline, higher pH level. You can also invest in full-home systems that will filter the water you shower or bathe in, as well as providing clean drinking water. Consider investing in an air filter as well, as there can be substantial indoor air pollution caused by the outgassing of chemicals used in the production of furniture, paint and carpets, as well as pet dander, bacteria and mould.

It should be obvious to consider smoking an absolute no-no, but in case you need a reminder, cigarettes contain known carcinogens and those who quit smoking after diagnosis have a higher overall survival.

Your cleaning products should be non-toxic and environmentally friendly. If they're friendly to the environment, they'll be friendly to you. Again, choose a trusted brand known for its environmental values and clean ingredients. Something you pick up in the supermarket labelled 'natural' may be far from it. Know your brands and buy wisely.

You'll be doing your pets a favour too. They walk on your freshly mopped floors or freshened-up carpets and then lick their feet, ingesting the chemicals directly. Keep yourself and your furry friends safe with more natural choices.

It can be difficult to avoid toxicity in furniture like sofas, due to regulations on flame retardants. However, if you have the option to avoid adding extra treatments like stain-resistance, that will help to reduce the toxic load in your home. If you want to get the biggest bang for your buck in reducing household toxicity, change your mattress for a non-toxic or organic one. Your bed is where you spend a large proportion of your time at home, so it's the area of greatest chemical exposure. Conventional mattresses tend to include toxic foams and glues, as well as flame-retardant chemicals, which are all outgassing as you sleep.

Review the soft furnishings you have in your home as well, opting for more natural, untreated fabrics. Consider the clothes you wear, and choose natural fibres over synthetics. Do what you can. It may not be financially viable to replace major items, but if you're making new purchases, bear your toxic load in mind.

The aim is to reduce the physical stress on your body, particularly while it's in the process of healing, not to create a new anxiety about needing to have a 100 per cent pure home environment. Every little choice you make to eat cleaner, avoid bottled water, choose natural body products, or opt for environmentally friendly household cleaners will help. Every small step is another stone in the foundation of your new practice of self-care – giving your body the nurturing it needs to heal.

Exercise

According to a 2017 *Canadian Medical Association Journal* review, being overweight at diagnosis increases the likelihood of a poorer prognosis, and gaining weight during or after treatment brings a higher risk of breast cancer-related death. However, the review also found that physical activity can reduce breast cancer mortality by about 40 per cent, and recommends around 150 minutes of exercise per week.[18]

No healing programme could be considered complete without adding exercise alongside dietary changes. For those of us who have had surgery, exercise options can be limited during recovery, but there are types of gentle exercise that work well for a body that may have restricted movement.

Walking is the obvious choice, and it's something that can be easily integrated into your day. The extra benefits of getting outdoors in nature also make it an excellent choice while you're healing. Swimming is another low-impact exercise option, but make sure your surgeon has confirmed that your wounds are sufficiently healed before diving into the pool or getting into a Jacuzzi, as you may run the risk of infection.

Chi Gong is a very gentle form of exercise that can help you to build up your stamina during treatment and increase your flexibility after surgery. Its postures come from martial arts and they follow the Traditional Chinese Medicine approach of building strength in the body's vital organs. Chi Gong's slow movements can be done standing or modified for sitting in a chair, so they can be adapted to suit whatever range of movement you're currently experiencing. Chi Gong has been found to have a positive effect on fatigue, the immune system and cortisol levels in cancer patients.[19]

Yoga has been my go-to exercise for recovering from three surgeries and regaining my range of movement after each one. There are slower forms of yoga that are ideal for the times when you're healing or going through treatment. If you're feeling exhausted but still need a stretch, restorative yoga is a fabulous choice. It focuses on allowing your body to relax into postures, supported by bolsters and blocks. There are only a few simple positions held during a restorative session, so it's slow-paced, meditative and very relaxing.

Yin yoga is my hands-down favourite form of yoga. Rather like restorative yoga, in yin yoga your body is supported by bolsters and blocks while you settle into a posture for around five minutes or so. With fewer postures than a normal yoga class and plenty of time to settle in to each one, it encourages you to listen to your body and never force a movement. While yin yoga is more active than restorative yoga, it's deeply meditative too, so you'll come out of a session not only feeling more flexible but also more at peace.

Supportive therapies

While you're healing, take the opportunity to treat yourself with supportive therapies you haven't tried before. I've used acupuncture throughout – regularly for general health maintenance and more intensely when recovering from surgery. I've also taken advantage of a local wellness centre offering taster sessions in everything from reflexology and reiki to sound healing and Indian head massage. Even during times when you can't lie comfortably to have a full oncology massage, you can find other small treatments or support sessions to give you a lift.

Oncology massage

Specialist oncology massage modifies techniques to safely work with the complications of cancer and cancer treatment. If you've had lymph nodes removed you can be at risk of lymphoedema, so make sure your therapist knows how to work with the lymphatic system to draw fluids away from the affected arm and breast area.

Breast Cancer Haven offers free counselling sessions at several centres across England, as well as therapies such as craniosacral, homeopathy, herbal medicine, hypnotherapy and aromatherapy. You can find your nearest location at www.breastcancerhaven.org.uk.

Maggie's Centres are drop-in clinics for cancer patients across the UK and in Hong Kong offering practical, emotional and social support, including stress management courses, exercise classes and expressive art sessions. See where they're located at www.maggiescentres.org.

Look for similar centres in your region. If there aren't any specific cancer-oriented clinics, you should be able to find wellness clinics that offer a range of nourishing complementary therapies.

A body changed by treatment

In your very natural rush to want to have the cancer removed, you may not have given much thought to what your body will look and feel like after surgery. Or that may be one of the issues that fills you with the greatest dread. Either way, cancer treatment leaves none of us as we were before – not on any level, and least of all on the physical one.

While the loss of your hair through chemotherapy is clearly devastating, losing a breast through mastectomy is a huge body blow to your sense of yourself as a woman. There is no easy way to say this – it's one of the hardest things you'll ever go through, not just the loss, but learning to live with the scarring and complete absence of a breast or breasts. Nothing anyone can say will ever make this anything less than horrific.

It doesn't matter that you believe it will save your life. A mastectomy strikes at the heart of your self-worth, your body image and your femininity. It unleashes an emotional pain like no other. And you must feel all of those feelings. Allow them to wash over you and be expressed – don't hide them inside. You'll cry buckets and that will help you heal.

There's just no sugar-coating this one. I can offer you help for easing the pain, but you can't avoid facing it. When you've had a chance to express and release your feelings, you'll be able to summon up that feisty feminine energy within you and get through it, putting one foot in front of the other, one day at a time.

Surgical scars

What I can give you is a view from the other side. In my first surgery – effectively a kind of lumpectomy combined with breast reduction and removal of lymph nodes – I was horrified by the smallest of scars. When I then went on to have a mastectomy, it showed me what scarring really was. And I lived with it for two and a half years before my reconstruction.

Slowly, slowly, I became accustomed to the changes in my body, and over time I watched them change from angry, red scars to thin, silver lines. While the seasons changed, the scars evolved. As I learned to make peace with my body as it was now – not how it had been – the scars were also beginning to fade. The small lymph node scar that I'd fixated on so much in the beginning isn't even visible these days.

My reconstruction scars are recent and quite dramatic – a huge train-track of a scar runs from hip to hip, my reconstructed breast has a Frankenstein-like line running across and underneath, and my reduced breast has a T-shape of scars running from the nipple to the suture line beneath it. Yet none of this even really bothers me now. Give it a year and it will fade. In two or three it will be barely noticeable.

This is the long game, and that's the one you need to play. No matter how unbearable it may seem in the moment, it will change. Your body does its healing work and you do your acceptance work. You're in partnership, and the only way out is through.

Wearing a breast prosthesis

Before leaving hospital after a mastectomy you'll usually be given a lightweight breast-shaped pad with a foam filling that sits inside your bra, to take the place of your breast. This is a stopgap measure until you have a fitting for a more solid breast prosthesis.

For women with smaller breasts, that first soft prosthesis is probably sufficient, but if you have larger breasts those pads are too light to take on the shape of a heavier breast, so you'll always look lopsided. A judiciously placed scarf will usually cover this up, until you can get an appointment to be measured for a silicone moulded prosthesis that's closer to your natural shape.

In the years when I had to wear a breast prosthesis, initially I felt very self-conscious about it and desperately wanted one that matched properly. Having waited months to get a silicone prosthesis, paradoxically I found it so heavy I barely used it. A surgeon once told me that's quite common, and that most women end up using the lightweight prosthesis in everyday life. Eventually I often found it more comfortable to leave the breast pad off altogether – apart from special occasions when I wanted a party dress to look natural.

> ### Breast prosthesis tips
>
> *You may have to adapt your personal style a little to keep your prosthesis from showing. Avoid low-cut or scoop neck tops or dresses, as it may be visible with these styles, or use a scarf to cover the neckline. You can buy mastectomy bras that have pockets for prostheses, plus you can find specially-designed swimsuits with those same pockets, as well as waterproof prostheses.*

Inner Smile meditation

When you're finding it hard to love your body and accept the changes it's going through, the Inner Smile meditation can help you to begin feeling kindly towards it. It comes from a Taoist approach to sending positive energy to your vital organs, but here we'll adapt it to send love to the places where your body has changed.

~ INNER SMILE MEDITATION ~

Practise this meditation regularly to bring you back into a more peaceful relationship with your body and to be more present to it. You could do it as a morning ritual before you get out of bed, and again at night to send you gently and peacefully into sleep.

1. Find a place where you can sit quietly for a few minutes. Sit cross-legged or in a chair with your feet on the floor, and place your hands in your lap. Start to breathe deeply and slowly, paying attention to how your breath feels as it moves through your body.

2. Feel as though your breath is moving right down into your hips as you inhale. When you have a gentle rhythm going, bring your attention to your heart. As you do so, think of something or someone you love, until you feel your heart fill up with joy and a smile rises to your face.

3. Now send that smile and that feeling of love to your scars and all the unloved places in your body. Smile to each place, one at a time, coming back to your loving heart and raising a new smile before you move onto the next. As you smile, send love and acceptance, feeling your body receive this positive energy.

4. When you've sent love to each of your scarred or unloved places, return to your heart and gather one last smile for your body as a whole. Start at the top of your head and shine your smile across your face and head, down your neck, across your shoulders, down your arms and torso and down your legs to your feet and toes.

5. Take a moment to notice how peaceful your body feels. Then gently wiggle your fingers and toes, and slowly bring yourself back to the room, opening your eyes.

~

Being comfortable in your body

Staying present to your body gives you access to your gut feelings and your intuition. We'll talk more about that in the section on mindfulness in Chapter 6, but in the meantime it can be helpful to create little rituals for yourself that put you in touch with your body throughout the day. A quick inner smile, a brief stretch routine, savouring the sunshine on your face or luxuriating in the scent of fresh flowers are all small ways to return to your senses. When you're present in your body, your focus moves out of your head and away from your worries.

Start to trust your body as a refuge again – a safe place to be. Focus on what it can do, not on what it has lost. Remember, there's a difference between being present and conscious in your body and being self-conscious about it. It's safe to inhabit your body. It's not letting you down. It's just trying to heal itself. You may be travelling through a vale of tears right now, but you won't be taking up residence there. Treating your body like a friend will help you navigate your way out.

For the times when your confidence in your appearance may be sagging, the international charity Look Good Feel Better can help. It offers workshops and online tutorials for women dealing with the side effects of cancer treatment. There are free in-person two-hour skincare and make-up sessions, as well as a range of online videos on wigs and headgear, plus cosmetic tips.

The Look Good Feel Better programme is run from locations in the UK, Ireland, Europe, the Middle East, Canada, USA, South America, Australia and New Zealand. It also offers a confidence kit by mail. Find your local office at www.lookgoodfeelbetter.co.uk/about/international/.

Embodiment checklist ✓

- Clean up your diet
- Reduce your toxic load
- Find exercise you enjoy
- Use supportive therapies
- Learn to accept your changed body

CHAPTER 5

Emotional Ease

Finding calm and letting go of the past

'Let difficulty transform you. And it will.
In my experience, we just need help in
learning how not to run away.'

Pema Chödrön

Nothing prepared me for how emotionally gruelling the experience of breast cancer could be. I'd had debilitating illnesses before, but this was next-level suffering. The fear of dying, the disfigurement, the endless hospital appointments and tests, the constant uncertainty – it all snowballs into your own personal hell.

Everything I'd learned in more than 30 years of spiritual practice gave me some solid ground to retreat to, but there were days when I could do nothing but cry. My go-to solution was to cry in the bath. There's something about the water that helps you to let go and have a proper sob. And the crying helps. When you let it all go and forget about trying to be brave, you're just your authentic self and there's an enormous relief in that. Tears don't wash away all the pain, but they do help you to let go of a lot of tension.

I'd always been a really private person, keeping my feelings to myself. Actually, I probably didn't even let myself feel them most of the time. Breast cancer opened the floodgates. I learned to be much more fluid with *my emotions and to let them flow through me, rather than damming them up. This brought me an enormous amount of peace, even in the toughest of times. I knew if I accepted the way that I felt and let it run its course, there would be a release and a rush of fresh energy afterwards.*

I let go of judgement about my emotions. I noticed them and felt them, but I didn't try to assess them, control them or limit them. I simply let them be. And they live much more on the surface for me now. They're more accessible and I'm much happier, more resilient and more peaceful.

Calm is a super power.

Not only does it let you ride the waves of your breast cancer experience without being sucked under by them, it also helps your body to heal.

Only when we're peaceful and at rest can our parasympathetic nervous system kick in to activate healing. When we're stressed, our sympathetic nervous system is in charge, and all our body's resources are focused outwards, activating the 'fight or flight' response. Any functions that are not essential are shut down. When the parasympathetic nervous system is active, it restores the body to a state of calm and is in charge of the 'rest and digest' functions of the body.

Because you're under a great deal of stress when you're trying to deal with breast cancer, the sympathetic nervous system becomes activated. Your adrenals are working overtime and your body is flooded with cortisol. This can keep you in a state of emotional panic and affect your ability to sleep when you need it most. It also adversely affects immune function, which is key to your recovery.

So how do you engage the parasympathetic nervous system? You slow down and induce your body into a more rested state. There are many simple techniques to help you do this, and the best starting place is your breath.

Breathing in calm

Firstly, pay attention to your breath. When you're stressed, your breathing pattern will be shorter and will stay higher in the chest. Try it now. Focus on your breath, keeping it shallow and high for a few seconds. Notice how you feel.

Now start to draw a longer breath, breathing deeper down into your lungs. Breathe more slowly again and bring it right down into your abdomen, feeling the rise and fall of your stomach as you take long inhalations and exhalations. For an even deeper and more grounding breath, imagine you're breathing right down into your hips. Notice how calm and present you feel.

Using your breath to manage your mood

Your breath is the gateway to changing how you feel. You can easily refresh yourself or calm yourself down by working with the length of your inhalation and exhalation. When you breathe out for longer than you

> *breathe in, you'll instantly feel more peaceful. When you reverse that balance and breathe in for longer than you breathe out, you'll feel energized.*
>
> *Use a four/eight count to get started, until you develop a rhythm. Breathe in for four and out for eight to calm yourself, or breathe in for eight and out for four when you need some extra energy.*
>
> *While you're waiting for a hospital appointment where you need to be alert to take in details, use a longer inhalation. If you're feeling fearful, use a longer exhalation to help yourself feel calm.*

Green is the new black

When you're feeling emotionally overwhelmed, being in nature can make an enormous difference to your mood. Going for a walk or simply sitting outside in the sunshine for a few minutes can give an instant boost to your flagging spirits. Setting aside a regular time to experience the healing power of the natural world can bring huge benefits.

In Japan, spending time in nature has been a key factor in preventative health care and healing since the 1980s. *Shinrin-yoku* or 'forest bathing' is practised by taking a gentle stroll in woodlands to immerse yourself in their sights, sounds and scents. It has been found to lower cortisol levels, elevate mood and improve immune function.

In a 2007 study by the Nippon Medical School in Tokyo, subjects taking two-hour walks in the woods over a two-day period showed a 50 per cent increase in their body's natural killer (NK) cells,[1] which are key players in immune response. A further study showed that the natural chemicals secreted by evergreen trees – wood essential oils known as phytoncides – were found to increase natural killer cell activity and the expression of anti-cancer proteins.[2]

Wherever you are, you can find simple ways to integrate the natural world into your life. Take a walk by the river, sit in a park, go to a botanical garden or find a forest or a lake for a day out. Enjoy nature with no agenda, staying present to the beauty around you, letting it heal and calm you. Leave your phone in your bag, turn off the ringer and keep your breath deep and slow. Even a few peaceful minutes outside can make a huge difference to your day.

Scents and sensibilities

Aromatherapy can be another powerful tool in your emotional balance arsenal. You can utilize its mood-altering powers in many ways, so enjoy getting creative with it. Carry an aromatherapy spray with you for an instantly uplifting spritz or use a lavender gel on your temples to soothe a worried mind. Try wearing a natural perfume with a fragrance that reminds you of happier times when you need a boost, soak in an essential oil bath to help you sleep or diffuse oils in your home to manage your moods.

The connection between fragrance and emotion isn't just an invention of the perfume companies. The scent receptors in our nose connect directly with the most ancient part of the brain, the limbic system, where our instinctive reactions reside. The sensations of smell are only relayed to our brain's 'thinking' cortex after more deep-seated emotional responses have been triggered.

Scent association is very personal. In the course of your life you'll build up a series of scent memories that create your own olfactory profile. Your childhood associations with scent will be carried with you throughout your life. Some will be conscious, others will not. You could have a deep aversion to a particular smell but may not recall the incident that triggered it.

Conversely, you could find yourself deeply attracted to a particular scent and may not be aware of why it's so powerful for you. And of course you can have very clear associations with people and events, like remembering the smell of your mother's perfume when she bent down to kiss you goodnight before going out for the evening.

When you're using aromatherapy to manage your moods, your personal preference is far more important than how effective a fragrance may be for other people. Even if someone else swears by it, a product will bring you no benefit if you dislike the scent. Equally, if you're going through chemotherapy, you may find yourself highly sensitive to scent, and aromatherapy products should be avoided while the sensitivity persists.

Essential oils for emotional ease

Here's a small selection of scents and the emotional states they support. You can diffuse essential oils in a room, add a few drops to a handkerchief to carry with you, buy a scented candle or mix some drops into a carrier oil and rub it around your neck and shoulders for a more lingering fragrance.

Uplifting

- *Bergamot will cheer you in dark times*

- *Cedarwood brings courage*

- *Frankincense is empowering*

- *Grapefruit offers optimism*

- *Juniper enhances your capacity for joy*

- *Lemongrass opens you up to new possibilities*

- *Neroli helps with clarity of choice*

- *Sweet orange invites light-heartedness*

- *Spikenard brings resilience*

- *Vetiver aids self-assurance*

- *Ylang-Ylang assists with mindfulness*

Calming

- *Chamomile is relaxing*

- *Cypress will help you feel supported*

- *Elemi brings serenity*

- *Lavender lets you feel nurtured*

- *Myrtle brings comfort*

- *Palmarosa invites self-compassion*

- *Patchouli induces peacefulness*

- *Pine assists with self-worth*

- *Rock Rose aids with shock and trauma*

- *Rose helps you to feel loved*

- *Sandalwood is grounding and contemplative*

Releasing negative emotions with EFT

Emotional Freedom Technique or EFT is an emotional healing technique based on the meridian system from Traditional Chinese Medicine. By focusing on a particular issue and tapping a sequence of acupuncture points on your body, you can reduce the emotional charge around an issue, calm your emotions and reduce fear. It can even help with the symptoms arising from hormonal therapies used to combat breast cancer.

The nine EFT tapping points are as follows:

1. Karate chop point on the side of the hand

2. Top of the head

3. Inside the eyebrow

4. Outside the eye

5. Beneath the eye

6. Underneath the nose

7. Beneath the lips

8. The collar bone

9. Under the armpit, roughly where your bra strap sits

This illustration shows the positions of the tapping points on the body. You can refer to it until you've memorized the sequence.

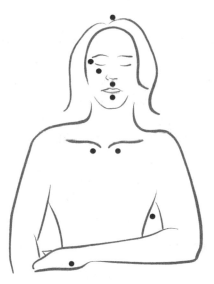

EFT tapping points

The basics of EFT tapping

To focus your healing, start by creating a two-part healing statement that reflects both how you feel now and how you would like to feel. For example, 'Even though I feel stressed and worried, I choose to relax and feel calm.'

You can use your healing statement to help with general feelings or specific events. For example you could say, 'Even though I have a hospital appointment today, I feel calm and in charge.' Or you can use it to help you overcome body issues that result from surgery, saying 'Even though my body is scarred, I choose to love and accept it.'

When you've chosen your healing statement, check in on the feeling you're trying to shake or situation you're concerned about, which is the first part of your statement. Give it a rating of 1–10 based on how negative or difficult it feels at the moment. This will give you a starting point, so that you can check in later to see how effective tapping has been for you.

Now try a couple of rounds of tapping. First, tap the karate chop point on your hand and work your way down your body through all nine points – beginning and ending at the karate chop point. Tap each point with your fingers as you say your full healing statement. After a couple of rounds, again ask yourself how you're feeling, and give that another 1–10 rating. If the negative or difficult feeling hasn't dissipated, keep doing rounds of tapping until you notice a shift.

To complete your EFT tapping session, do a couple more rounds using just the second part of your healing statement that expresses how you want to feel, like 'I feel calm and in charge' or 'I love and accept my body.' You can practise

EFT on any issue that comes to mind. It could be something small that crops up in your daily experience or it could be a long-standing emotional issue.

Physical symptoms can also be affected with the use of EFT. In a 2014 study by Baker & Hoffman published in the *European Journal Of Integrative Medicine*,[3] EFT was used to manage the side effects associated with tamoxifen and aromatase inhibitors in women with breast cancer. These drugs block the body's production of oestrogen, and create menopausal side effects. Participants in the study received a three-week course in EFT and used it for the following nine weeks. Statistically significant improvements were noted in total mood disturbance, anxiety, depression and fatigue – and the number of hot flushes decreased.

EFT is also now used by many trauma therapists to work with patients suffering from post-traumatic stress disorder (PTSD). This leads us on to the big opportunity that breast cancer brings – releasing old pain to accelerate healing.

How trauma affects your health

To fully understand how your emotions affect your body, you have to go right back to your earliest years. The CDC-Kaiser Permanente Adverse Childhood Experiences Study commissioned by the US Centers for Disease Control and Prevention (CDC) was published in 1998, and was the first to link adverse childhood experiences (ACEs) with a lifetime of ensuing health issues, including heart disease, cancer and many autoimmune diseases.

Three different categories of trauma were measured in the ACE study – abuse, household challenges and neglect. Abuse included emotional, physical or sexual abuse. Household challenges were exposure to violent treatment of the mother, substance abuse, mental illness, parental separation or divorce, or having a criminal household member. Neglect included both emotional neglect and physical neglect. Each type of trauma experienced was tallied to create an ACE score.[4]

As you can see, what we often think of as quite a normal experience – emotional neglect – is considered to be a trauma. Intensity is also a consideration. If you experienced toxic stress over extended periods as a child, this is likely to increase the risk to your long-term health.

The CDC describes the progression of possible consequences from ACEs as a pyramid, with ACEs at the foundation, leading to disrupted neurodevelopment, which can manifest as social, emotional and cognitive impairment. That impairment is fertile ground for the adoption of health-risk behaviours, which in turn can lead to disease, disability and social problems, with a potential outcome of early death.[5]

I'm sharing this with you so you'll understand how disease can be an outcome of ACEs, but please don't let it scare you. The ACE pyramid shows a likely progression, but it's not carved in stone. It doesn't take into account any form of intervention or healing, which is what you're going to find out about next. The good news is coming up soon.

Here's the science bit – concentrate!

Trauma affects your body's physiology. When you experience it, your brain's fear centre – the amygdala – sounds the alarm and responds with a series of hormonal and physiological changes. Your sympathetic nervous system goes into 'fight, flight or freeze' mode and shuts down all non-essential body and brain functions.

Normally, when the threat has passed, the parasympathetic nervous system will kick in and restore the body to its usual functioning. But for many trauma survivors, this doesn't happen and the body stays on high alert. The amygdala keeps looking for threats and the hippocampus can be underdeveloped, making it difficult to distinguish between past and present memories. The ventromedial prefrontal cortex shrinks and diminishes the capacity to regulate emotions, and the body's ability to regulate itself is impaired. This toxic soup fatigues the body and many of its systems.

The relatively recent science of psychoneuroimmunology (PNI) studies the interaction between the body's psychological processes and its nervous and immune systems. Its studies have also found a strong correlation between stress and impairment of immune function.

Finally, some good news. The Somatic Experiencing® techniques developed by leading traumatologist Peter Levine are a body-based pathway that can help to reverse the impact of trauma. And the science of epigenetics shows that while gene function can be impaired or switched off by environmental factors – physical, mental and emotional – gene expression can also be switched back on.

The effort we put in to healing our traumas will pay off in altered gene expression and its knock-on effect on our health. When we work with trauma and our habitual stress response, we're influencing our biochemistry positively and enhancing our physical wellbeing.

Emotional healing supercharges wellness

We know that our untreated trauma – or even something as simple as a long-held resentment – can have a physiological effect, so just like having a spring clean in a dirty house, we need to investigate our old wounds in order to release them. When we do this, we support the body in its healing process.

Getting professional help

Before we begin looking at ways to shift old emotional issues, consider doing this in tandem with a professional. If you have PTSD or deep-seated emotional problems, you will need the support of a trained therapist.

If that is the case, do not try to go it alone. If you're severely traumatized, you can run the risk of re-traumatizing yourself without the necessary professional support. If at any point you find yourself deeply distressed, focus on your body sensations to return yourself to an awareness of the present moment, and seek therapeutic help straight away.

Feeling our feelings, unravelling our stories

For every trauma we've experienced, there are two parts. There are the facts of what happened and also what we told ourselves that the incident meant – about others and about ourselves.

Imagine you're rejected by your first love. Your emotions run deep and of course it's devastating. All of that is true. But then your mind steps in and begins to build a story around it. *He didn't love me because I'm not pretty enough. My breasts are too small. My thighs are too big. I wasn't smart or funny enough.*

These repetitive thoughts can soon degenerate into deeply held beliefs that are more wide-ranging and damaging, like *I'm unlovable, No man will ever want me* or *I'm unlucky in love.* These beliefs then become our immutable truths. The reality is that one man rejected us, and we now believe that *all* men will reject us – or any variation on that theme.

To unlock the energy that's trapped in these stories, we must first feel the intensity of the feelings that we avoided when the event occurred, and then ask what that made us believe about ourselves. When we allow the depth of our pain to be felt without resisting it, we can begin to move through to more clarity about the event, and loosen the stories we've built up around it.

It's important to feel your feelings as much as you can, so you can wade through the overwhelming emotions to get to the release on the other side of them. We tend to avoid pain, and yet the avoidance of it keeps the emotions stuck. Paradoxically, it's often more painful to stay in fear of our emotional intensity than to simply experience it and let it go.

When you have an issue that you're ready to deal with, try this exercise. Don't go headlong into the worst trauma you've ever experienced. Start with something simple, like a recent rejection at work, a time when someone made you feel shame for being who you are, or a relationship breakup that was upsetting but not devastating.

~ EMOTIONAL HEALING INNER DIALOGUE ~

Sit quietly and comfortably somewhere where you won't be disturbed, and gently work through these steps, giving yourself plenty of time to experience the full intensity of your feelings.

1. Close your eyes and begin breathing deeply, right down into your hips. When your breathing has a deep, steady rhythm, imagine that you have a grounding cord growing out of your tailbone and feel it travel down beneath you, right to the centre of the Earth. Secure your cord there, perhaps to a rock or a crystal, and feel yourself safe and grounded

2. Imagine light coming up from that secure point, through your body and up out through your head into the sky. And feel light travelling down from the sky above you – through your body and down into the Earth below. Feel the safety and support of this stream of light as it flows through you.

3. Now bring to mind a specific event related to the issue you want to work with. See it unfold before you and begin to feel the feelings that it brings up. Experience how it made you feel in that moment, and let your emotions flow. Take your time and don't reject any feeling, however uncomfortable it may make you. Stay with it until the emotions lighten.

4. See the main person or group of people who were part of that event in front of you. Tell them how it made you feel. Tell them all the stories you've told yourself since then about the meaning that event had for you. Don't hold back. Let yourself express your deepest fears about what it means about you. Again, stay with it until you feel like you've said everything you need to say.

5. If you want to, you can ask them why they did what they did, and listen for an answer. If you don't feel comfortable, you can move onto the next step, but this can be a crucial part of forgiveness and release – not to make what they did right, but to understand why. There may not be a reason. They may simply not have considered their impact on you. But that is an answer in itself – they didn't have the emotional capacity to understand how they affected you.

6. When you feel complete with that discussion, it's time for some energetic healing. Let the hurt that you've felt take on a shape and appear in the air in front of you. It could be any kind of shape – a flower, a ball of light, whatever you like. It's there to take on any emotional stress or darkness still left in your body.

7. See the pain and the stories appear like dark smoke, leaving your body and filling up the shape. As each shape becomes

full, send it up into the sky where it will explode like a firework and disappear. Keep filling up the shapes and releasing them until you feel a sense of completion. When you're ready, feel yourself surrounded by beautiful golden light, healed and restored.

8. Come back to the room slowly, first wiggling your fingers and toes, and then opening your eyes. Feel the sense of release now that the old stories have left you and you can appreciate the truth about yourself, not the tales your mind made up.

~

Make sure to drink plenty of water after this inner dialogue and give yourself time to integrate the healing. Don't rush into activity or connect with other people until you feel ready. Emotional healing can be tiring and leave you feeling sensitive, so be compassionate with yourself and keep things low-key for as long as you need. You can repeat this healing whenever you need to release emotions, and use the process for any painful event in your life.

Healing and forgiveness

A huge part of healing is forgiveness, and that's a very misunderstood word. We're often reluctant to forgive because we think that forgiveness lets someone off the hook for their actions. But forgiveness isn't about condoning bad behaviour or giving someone a 'get out of jail free' card. It's a letting go. It's setting yourself free from what happened to you – free from carrying the pain of someone else's actions.

We forgive them to free ourselves. We look beyond what they did, so we can release ourselves from bondage.

Forgiveness isn't just for the other person's sake. It's a gift we give to ourselves. If you're struggling to forgive someone, try saying that you release them instead. It's a trick of the mind, but it will help to set you free from emotional pain.

And don't forget to forgive yourself. When something traumatic has happened to us, we so often blame ourselves. Even if it happened when we were very young, and we consciously know it wasn't our fault, there can still be a level of self-blame to be released. Forgive yourself for all the ways you made it your fault, and all the self-attack you've put yourself through. Be compassionate with yourself so you can release the pain that's keeping you stuck in the past.

As we talked about earlier, if you want to work with more deep-seated trauma it's best to work with a professional. However, traumatologist Peter Levine has developed some simple exercises you can do at home. This one will help you to feel safe when emotions are running high.

~ SELF-HOLDING ~

When you feel scattered, frightened or fractious, this exercise can help you to settle in comfortably within the boundaries of your body. Peter Levine says that 'the body is the container of all of our sensations and all of our feelings. When the person can feel the container, then the emotions and sensations do not feel as overwhelming because they are contained.'

1. Cross your arms in front of you, as though you're giving yourself a hug. Allow yourself to settle into the position, feeling supported and contained.

2. Notice if anything changes in your breathing or the sensations in your body. Simply pay attention and notice how you feel.

3. Sit with it for a while, until you feel a sense of relief. The goal here is to feel safe in your body, and to allow emotional ease.

~

Discover more of Peter Levine's work in his books *Healing Trauma*, *Waking The Tiger* and *In An Unspoken Voice*.

Emotional bandwidth

Breast cancer is a trauma in itself. While you're going through it, you'll have a lot of intense emotions to deal with and you'll need both the privacy and support to do that. This is your opportunity to finally take charge of your time and energy, and to set aside your natural reaction to respond to others' needs.

Being on an emotional rollercoaster is exhausting. You will find it hard to achieve as much as you normally do. Even a single hospital appointment may leave you feeling deflated and fatigued for the rest of the day or even for days afterwards.

If you want to keep your energy high, you must consider your emotional bandwidth and who affects it. The people you allow closest to you need to be the ones who are the most supportive and the least judgemental. At a time when stress makes you feel extra thin-skinned, the tribe you want to gather around you are the cheerleaders, the caring ones, the fun people and the helpers.

Think of yourself as a planet with moons orbiting around you. The ones in the closest orbit are those who put the least pressure on you and offer practical support. The ones who need to be shifted into your outer orbit are the draining ones, the needy types, the opinionated ones and anyone who places expectations on you. You don't know how you're going to feel on any given day, so your friends need to be flexible and understanding.

When you're dealing with a life-threatening situation, a lot becomes clear. You won't have patience for silly dramas and squabbles. You've got a big enough drama going on in your own life. You won't have patience for pretence either. Life has become very real. And you're very grateful for the life you have. Every moment counts. You won't want to waste it.

Choose your companions carefully, give only the time and energy that you can freely give and only commit to what you want to do – never do anything out of duty. Those days are over. You're becoming more emotionally authentic than ever before. Don't abandon yourself for someone else's priorities. You need every ounce of energy you can muster for your own journey.

You'll want time on your own to process your thoughts and feelings. Your life depends on it. Don't feel guilty. There will be time enough for everyone else later. For the moment, it's about you. Make yourself your priority. Give yourself shameless self-care.

Now that we've calmed the emotional waves, we're going to take a look at how to deal with the mental stress of dealing with breast cancer, and how having a tranquil mind helps you with your treatment choices.

Emotional ease checklist ✓

- Control your breath to manage your mood
- Spend time outdoors for the healing power of nature
- Use therapeutic scents to calm and uplift you
- Release negative emotions with EFT
- Overcome past trauma with emotional healing
- Learn what helps you to comfort yourself
- Practise forgiveness to free yourself from emotional pain
- Manage your emotional bandwidth

CHAPTER 6

Clarity of Mind

Easing fear and making good choices

*'You must learn a new way to think before
you can master a new way to be.'*

MARIANNE WILLIAMSON

Going into my second breast cancer surgery after the first one failed, I felt like the White Queen in Through the Looking-Glass – *the sequel to* Alice's Adventures in Wonderland – *who lived her life backwards. I was feeling the pain before it happened.*

The first surgery had been terrifying enough, but it was one intended to save as much of my breast as possible – in effect, a breast reduction. The second surgery was a mastectomy. Nothing would be left. And I had a month and a half to live with my scarred Frankenbreast before it would be gone forever. I was forced into a curious grieving process, saying a long goodbye to a part of my body I would never see again.

Losing a breast somehow felt shameful. I didn't want anyone to know, but as a large-breasted woman it was difficult to disguise. Scarves and loose clothing quickly became my best friends, as I struggled with a temporary prosthesis that was woefully inadequate in size and shape. Getting dressed as a one-breasted Amazon is a daily reminder of breast cancer. You never have the chance to put it behind you. You just have to learn to live with it.

And you learn how fragile your sense of femininity can be. When you have a 50 per cent deficit in the breast department, you're not guaranteed to feel sexy. Far from it. More likely you'll feel disfigured and have doubts about ever feeling attractive again. This is where attitude is everything.

Mindfulness may seem like the latest buzzword, but it is powerful medicine. Staying in the present moment will save you a lot of pain as you navigate your choices, adjust to your changing energy levels, deal with fear, and learn to embrace the impact of surgery.

When you're diagnosed with cancer, you're not just dealing with your own personal experience of it. You're dealing with a collective belief about the disease that is so ingrained it's barely conscious. And that belief is terrifying – cancer could kill you. Even if you're diagnosed at an early stage and your cancer is treatable, overwhelming fear is an instinctive response. As cancer patients, we need to learn how to self-soothe when fear arises, because it will. And often. It's a very understandable and very human response. There's nothing logical about fear.

Being mindful, staying in the moment

Only when we can mindfully separate our fears from our actual experience can we learn to calm ourselves and cultivate a clear mind. Fear can drive us into making serious life choices without considering the ramifications. It can keep us in an endless loop of second-guessing our options, so we're afraid to move forwards. And just as importantly, it turns on our 'fight or flight' response that stops our parasympathetic nervous system from kicking in and helping us to heal when we need it most.

Fear is the real villain in the breast cancer story. When your body is sick and struggling to perform its natural self-protective function, your mind – fuelled by the negative cultural narrative around cancer – will run rampant, indulging in every worst-case scenario it can conjure.

This 'awfulizing' is the most destructive thing you can do to yourself. If you're already being challenged on every level – emotionally, physically, mentally and spiritually – the last thing you need is self-attack. You must learn to train your mind to be your friend, not to tell you ghost stories that terrify you in the middle of the night. You can develop the power to discern what's important, what's true and what's really worth your concern.

Worry is fear's closest friend. While some fears may be realistic, worry is fear dressed up as something useful. When we worry, we feel like we're doing something constructive, when all we're actually doing is scaring ourselves. It gives us the illusion of purpose, but achieves nothing.

The best and most straightforward advice on worry comes from Stephen Spielberg's Cold War movie, *Bridge of Spies*. As a suspected Soviet spy who remains calm when facing a possible death sentence for espionage, Mark Rylance's character is asked by his lawyer, played by Tom Hanks, 'Do you never worry?

His response is simple. 'Would it help?'

Mindfulness means living in the present, moment by moment. When you have breast cancer, that's the safest place to be. There's so much uncertainty when cancer enters your life – you start living from appointment to appointment and test to test. The future feels bleak when your mind gets into the habit of awfulizing and creating endless worst-case scenarios.

But all that turmoil is for naught – your mind doesn't have the answers and you don't know the outcome. Anything is possible when you take charge of your healing, so the kindest way to deal with a rampaging mind is to bring it back to exactly where you are right now.

The present moment – your haven

When you're being swept into the whirlwind of constant activity, decision-making and other people's opinions, your place of safety is the present moment. However dark tomorrow may feel, in the here and now you are safe.

Take a deep, slow breath and remind yourself that you're OK. In this moment, you're safe. Focus for a moment on the practical things. You have a roof over your head, food in the fridge and the love of family and friends. For now, this is enough. For now, in this moment, rest in the safety that surrounds you. Breathe it in, feel the love, and feel the ground solid beneath you.

Gratitude as a quick mood shift

If you're feeling anxious, pay attention to your physical sensations, so you're drawing yourself back to the experience of being in your body, not lost in your head. This will ground you and allow you to move from panic and overwhelm back into a calmer and more centred state.

When you begin to feel more relaxed, if your mood needs more of a lift, start to think of all the things in your life that you're grateful for – a happy home, a beloved pet, good friends, a beautiful garden or sunny days. When your mind is out of control, you first need to calm it down, and then throw the dog a bone. Your mind will always want something to focus on, so it might as well be something good. Use an affirmation if that resonates with you. It's often easier to simply repeat a phrase over and over as a mantra when you're feeling stressed, rather than trying to conjure up more complex images in your mind. Start with something simple like 'In this moment I'm safe and at peace.'

Create your own personal mantra that helps you return to a feeling of safety. The more you use it, the more it will be anchored in your body, and you'll naturally start to relax when you say it. Get creative and expand your repertoire, so you have a mantra for every occasion. One of Louise Hay's favourite ones that works well for hospital visits and treatments is 'All hands that touch me are healing hands.' If you're having a wobble, try 'I'm in control of my healing' or 'My immune system is strong and knows how to heal itself.'

Making choices

The amount of information you'll be bombarded with and the new learning you will go through when breast cancer enters your life is staggering. You'll be flooded with medical details about your condition that will seem like an entire new language you have to learn, and the options for treatment are countless. You will be making decisions every day that will have far-reaching effects on your life, often when you feel completely unprepared to make them.

This is where mindfulness is your friend. When you learn to step back, calm your fears and find some space between your thoughts, you can tune in to your own powerful inner knowing. If you're in a panic, you'll go around in mental circles and won't be able to feel into what's right for you.

Ever had a day that started out badly, sent you into a tailspin and ended up even worse? In Traditional Chinese Medicine that fractious energy where you feel totally panicked is called 'reckless chi'. Learn to recognize its energy signature. When you feel reckless chi rising, you're cutting yourself off from your own internal guidance system. To think clearly and make the decisions that are right for you, you need to be calm and centred. If you're trying to make a decision that rings true to you, you need to be present in your body.

You've already learned how mindfulness helps to bring you back to an awareness of your body and to self-soothe, reducing the panic. When your mind is calmer, you'll be in a state where you can start to make authentic and empowered decisions. Do not fall for false urgency. You can take the time you need to make important medical decisions. If your doctor wants an answer on the spot, ask to take an afternoon or day to think about it and then phone back with your response. Don't let anyone else's agenda take precedence over your own.

After you've done your research on the options available to you, if you're still not absolutely clear on which way to go, pick two and start to feel into them. Before you do this, make sure you're somewhere where you feel calm and relaxed, and won't be disturbed. Think of your first option, then start to notice any changes of sensation in your body. You might find that you stay relaxed or you may find that your throat tightens or you get a sick feeling in your stomach.

The indicators of your gut instinct are very personal. Your job is just to notice how you feel as you think of this option and not to analyse it. Pay attention, and even jot down a few notes if that helps. Then spend a minute or two just being present with your surroundings before you move on to your second option. Again, notice the sensations that arise in your body as you think about going ahead with that option. You're not trying to weigh up the pros and cons. You're simply trying to get a sense of how it feels.

Come back to the present moment again, perhaps taking a few deep breaths, and start to compare how they felt. You should have a clear indication of which one felt more positive than the other. If there's not much difference between them, try the Two Roads meditation to get a deeper sense of what will work for you.

~ TWO ROADS MEDITATION ~

This guided meditation will help your imagination bypass your analytical thoughts, so you can feel a stronger instinct towards one of two options.

1. Sit quietly in a place where you won't be disturbed, with your feet on the ground and hands held loosely in your lap. Take some long, slow, deep breaths, breathing down deep into your body, right down into your hips, until you feel relaxed and serene.

2. In your mind's eye, see yourself walking through a green and sunny landscape, until a gently meandering path opens up before you. Walk on for a while, noticing how beautiful the flowers and trees are and how warm your body feels in the sun, with a gentle breeze caressing your face.

3. Then, in the distance, you see that the path is coming to an end, at a point where two roads diverge. When you reach that point, you'll see a signpost with your first option pointing in one direction and your second option in the opposite direction.

4. Take the first road and start to walk down it, again noticing the details around you. After walking for a little while, pay attention to how the landscape changes. Is it suddenly greener or rockier or are there more hills? Is the road straighter or more crooked? Does the weather change? Is it warmer or cooler? Are there more animals in this landscape compared to the path you first walked on?

5. When you have a sense of this landscape, turn around and walk back down the road to the signpost. Look back at the path that brought you here and remind yourself how beautiful it was.

Then set off down the second road, walking for a short while before you start to look for changes in the landscape, the light, the temperature or the wildlife around you.

6. When you feel you have a clear sense of this road, turn back and head for the signpost again. Once there, set off on your original path until you feel completely relaxed and happy.

7. When you're ready, return your attention to the room, gently wiggling your fingers and toes to bring yourself back to your body. You should instantly have a strong and clear feeling about which road felt brighter and easier, giving you a clear direction on which choice is right for you.

~

Once you've made your choices, don't second-guess them. If new information becomes available, of course you need to be open to that, but generally if you've made a decision, stick to it. You can drive yourself mad if you keep going over the same ground again and again.

That brings us to the cyclical nature of thought. We all have mental grooves that we've carved over years of repetitive thought. A large proportion of them will be grooves of self-attack. Those are the ones where we berate ourselves for not being smart enough, not doing something properly or for believing we've got this handled. Those thoughts won't ever entirely go away, but you can learn to manage them and introduce more positive grooves. Having thought patterns that nourish you may be a complete revelation to you if you've lived most of your life attacking yourself.

Mindfulness comes to the rescue for persistent thought grooves too. It's going to be a very handy tool in your breast cancer recovery toolkit. To break negative thought cycles, you have to notice that they exist in the first place. Initially, you may just realize that you're feeling frightened and depressed about your future, without isolating the thoughts that lie beneath that.

Don't worry, that's a starting point. Keep paying attention and you'll recognize the subjects that your mind returns to again and again. Then it becomes a mindful choice about where you want to direct your attention, rather than simply allowing your negative thoughts to run riot.

Overcoming persistent fears

Breast cancer is an opportunity to bring new awareness to how you're living your life. It invites you to examine your habitual ways of being and thinking. You can change your patterns, but first you need to develop a habit of observing them.

Going through treatment is a stressful time, but you can learn to bring yourself back to a state of peace and calm when you pay attention to how you're feeling throughout the day. If you start to feel out of sorts, notice which thoughts have been running around in your head. You'll tend to find that they are repetitive, and there are ones that you keep returning to. Usually they will focus on a frightening future or mistakes of the past.

To help you shift those grooves, it can be useful to give that repetitive voice a personality and a name. That way you can thank it for sharing and move on to a more positive train of thought. Give the voice a name that makes you laugh and reminds you of a Debbie Downer kind of person, always moaning. This will allow you to create a sense of separation between you and your thoughts and bring in a little humour.

As you go through your day, pay attention to how your mood shifts and changes. As it does, notice the thought grooves that accompany those shifts. Are they fears of the future – not surviving, being disfigured by surgery or suffering the side effects of treatment? Or are they coming from the past – blaming yourself for having the disease, or feeling lonely or unlovable?

A challenge as big as breast cancer will bring up all your most self-defeating beliefs, and your fears will loom larger than ever. Your work in the healing process is to release yourself from that old patterning, and take control of your thoughts, putting all your energy into creating a healthy mind, body and spirit.

When you can become aware of your thought grooves, your mind becomes a healing tool, not a destructive one. When future fears come up, acknowledge their presence, but move on to creating a new, more positive line of thought. You can self-soothe those fears with thoughts of how you're taking an active role in your healing and giving yourself the best possible chance to recover.

For persistent worries, remind yourself that in this moment you're safe and you're healing. Think of all the love and support that surrounds you. Imagine your healing team surrounding you with their loving care, gently nursing you back to wellness.

Quieting the inner critic

If the voice in your head is a self-critical one, it's building on the pain of the past to torture you with new scenarios of inadequacy. Those issues already existed, but now fear is magnifying them. That critical voice may come up with thoughts of how no-one will find you attractive with all the body changes you're going through, or that you should have taken better care of yourself.

To manage this voice, it helps to listen to what it's saying and respond objectively. Is it really true? What are the facts? Millions of people go through treatment every year and they still find or maintain romantic relationships, and breast cancer is a disease caused by myriad factors that you couldn't possibly have predicted.

When you can take some of the power out of the critical voice's accusations, you can move on to more helpful trains of thought. Try saying, *I choose to love myself as I am, and allow love in* or *I did the best I could with what I knew at the time, and now I'm taking charge of my healing.*

Consider this your daily practice. At first it may feel unnatural to be observing your thoughts, but if you persevere you'll begin to notice recurrent negative patterns. As you notice them, you can disempower them and turn your mind to creating thought grooves that support your healing.

Self-soothing for your inner child

Inside all of us are parts that are less developed than others. No matter how accomplished we are or how strong we may feel, underneath all our confidence in the world there still lies a frightened little girl who will appear when we're under the greatest threat. When we're feeling overwhelmed and at our most disheartened, we're expressing the fears and helplessness of that inner child.

~ COMFORTING YOUR INNER CHILD MEDITATION ~

Learning to soothe your inner child can bring you great comfort in the most difficult of times. Use this meditation when mindfulness feels like too much of an effort and you simply need some comfort.

1. Sit quietly in a peaceful place where you won't be disturbed. Make sure your feet are on the ground and your hands are held loosely in your lap.

2. Begin to breathe deeply. Lengthen your exhale to slow your breathing, and inhale all the way down into your hips. As you feel yourself relax, see yourself as a small girl in your mind's eye.

3. Notice how she seems and what she's doing.

4. Begin a conversation with her and ask her how she is feeling. Find out what's bothering her. Ask her what would help her to feel better. See yourself giving her whatever she needs. If she's

happy to have you come closer, hold her hand or let her sit on your lap so you can comfort her. Feel yourself giving your love to her, and watch how she changes.

5. Take all the time she needs to feel comforted, and when you're both ready, promise her that you'll always take care of her. Place her gently in your heart, telling her to call for you when she needs you, letting her know that you will always be there for her.

6. Bring your attention back to your surroundings, gently moving your fingers and toes to wake up your body, and return to the room.

~

Don't underestimate the power of this simple meditation. As you develop a relationship with your inner child, you'll not only learn to self-soothe, but she will start to remind you what's missing from your life. She may ask for more play, more fun, more time for yourself, or to explore your creativity. Be open to her suggestions and put them into practice. She's a part of you that knows what she needs to feel safe and secure, and she's a gateway to expressing your authentic self.

Journaling

Another way of releasing worries and finding some headspace is to write. Some people like to blog their healing stories as they happen, and others prefer to keep their experiences private while they're undergoing them.

You'll know what suits you best. You may never go public with your story, but writing is a healing process that can help you release anxieties and express feelings you may not feel comfortable sharing with others.

Julia Cameron's wonderful book on the creative process, *The Artist's Way*, introduces the idea of Morning Pages to help creativity flow and to keep a clear mind. She recommends journaling three pages each morning of free-flowing mind chatter. In this writing exercise, you're not trying to construct or tell a story, but just downloading what's in your head.

When you're in the maelstrom of rollercoaster emotions, constant uncertainty and time-sucking medical appointments, writing three pages every morning can be a big ask. To make it easier to fit in with so many demands on your time and energy, I've adapted this to a single Morning Page, to do a quick brain dump. That's all you have to commit to, and if you want to do more, you can.

Just take your journal and write a page in the morning of whatever's on your mind. Don't censor it, or try to make it sound pretty. Let petty irritations come out, big emotions, and nagging fears. There's no need to read it back. Its job is to remove the interference of niggling thoughts, so you'll have a clearer mind to start the day.

Over time, you'll get guidance from the pages you're writing, because common themes will come up. If you go beyond a single page, you'll find your mind will wander past the first level of thought into a more inspirational phase. You can explore that at your leisure. When you're in the trenches with treatments or recovery from surgery, just try to get that single page done. It will keep you sane.

Indulge your 'guilty pleasures'

Actually, there's no such thing as a guilty pleasure. There should be no shame in flipping through magazines, watching made-for-TV movies or reading trashy novels. While you're healing you won't have a great deal of concentration and you need to keep your mind occupied to keep it away from worry.

Now is not the time to force yourself to make highbrow choices. If you love a good afternoon movie on TV, go for it. Want to read a celeb-obsessed mag for a laugh? Do it. If it takes your mind off what you're going through, it's a good choice. Be kind to yourself and keep it fun and light.

The Aliveness Oracle

For really bad days, it helps to have a resource to remind you what makes you feel alive. When you look in the mirror and all you see is a tired and stressed woman looking back at you, you'll need a reminder that feeling good again is a possibility. On those days, you'll be short of imagination, energy and inspiration, so use your better days to create a legacy for the ones that aren't so good.

I call this the Aliveness Oracle. It's a collection of activities and experiences that delight you, amuse you, or revive your energy that you can tap into when you need a boost. When you can't even remember what happy felt like, your personal oracle will act as a reminder of the small moments that lift your spirit. Here's how you can make one of your own.

~ CREATING AN ALIVENESS ORACLE ~

The way you create your oracle is up to you. If you're a high-tech kind of woman, you can create it as an online mind map or as a list on your phone's Notes app. If you prefer putting pen to paper, you can brainstorm your ideas in a notebook and then transfer them to individual index cards.

Even better, get some blank cards and go to town with collaging images and inspirational words. Beauty and creativity uplift the spirit, so have fun with this and make your oracle something that lights you up whenever you see it.

1. First, come up with ideas for at least a dozen experiences that make you feel alive. These activities should range from small things you can do at home with little effort for recovery days to ones that require you to connect with others or venture out when you're feeling more energetic.

2. Each experience should be something that lifts your heart and puts you in touch with your aliveness. It could be as simple as having a special coffee or calling a friend, buying fresh flowers, taking a walk in nature, having a bubble bath, listening to an uplifting podcast, watching your favourite film or going to an art gallery. You know what your indulgences are. If buying a new lipstick puts a smile on your face, add that to the list. Nothing is too shallow or too silly. This is about having fun and feeling the life force within you.

3. When you're feeling flat, treat your mind map or activity cards like an oracle – pick one and do it. Keep expanding the oracle as you begin to heal, so your options become increasingly adventurous and bring you more in touch with the life you truly want to live. A compelling vision of the life you want to lead after cancer will pull you through even the darkest hours.

~

Let's stop here for just a moment to get in touch with that vision of life beyond breast cancer. Take a deep breath and imagine what an ideal day might look like for you. Visualize every detail of how you want to feel – vibrant, healthy, joyful, connected and on purpose. See yourself doing the things you love to do.

Start with how you wake up. Think of your plans for the day, experience them as though they're happening and see yourself going to sleep peacefully and delighted at how well the day turned out.

This is the vision that will get you to the other side. Think of what and who you have to live for. Wake up that aliveness and zest for life that's sleeping right now. Use your oracle to remind you of this every day.

~ ALIVENESS MEDITATION ~

If you're running on empty and losing sight of ever feeling well again, here's a quick meditation to get you in touch with your sense of aliveness and wellness again.

1. Sitting quietly, breathe deeply until you feel your body relax and your mind become quieter.

2. As you breathe, bring your attention to your heart and notice how it feels. You can bring your hand to your heart if it helps you to bring your attention there. Inhale deeply into your heart, and sense the aliveness that lives there. It might only feel like a small flicker at first, but notice how it grows.

3. Sense your heart as the fiery core of your being, pumping blood around your body, bringing wellness to every cell. As you do this, bring to mind the things you love – people, places, animals, art, music and experiences.

4. Feel how each one adds to that fiery sense of aliveness in your heart – as though your heart is overflowing with flames of joy, and that heat is spreading throughout your body, warming you with its love.

5. When the feeling of having your heart on fire is so strong that you're bursting with happiness, bring that energy back with you as you gently return to the room, feeling juicy, alive and inspired.

~

As you become more adept at managing your thoughts, you'll find yourself becoming more resilient when dealing with others' unintended insensitivities. Mindfulness will help you deal calmly with those who want to challenge you on your approach or tell you other people's breast cancer horror stories. Breast cancer and childbirth are two times in a woman's life when she's guaranteed to hear the worst stories about the experience precisely when she doesn't need to hear them. Becoming mindful will help you to understand your needs and communicate them effectively to others too.

A word on setbacks

When it comes to setbacks, where you place your attention will have a dramatic effect on your mood, your sense of safety and how your body copes with stress. However positive you may feel, things don't always go to plan. There may be more surgery, longer treatment or a worse prognosis than you expected.

My longed-for reconstructive surgery was postponed just as I was about to go into theatre. I'd stayed in hospital overnight, the surgeon had marked me up, and we were all ready to roll when we discovered that the anaesthetist had been called away to an emergency. It was a huge blow at the time, as I had already waited for more than two years for the surgery.

That ride home from the hospital was hell, but I had a mini-meltdown for a day or so and then started looking for things to do that I couldn't have done if the surgery had gone ahead. Opening up to new opportunities gave the setback a purpose. That's resilience. It's not false positivity. You feel the blows, allow your emotions to run their course and then you move on. You find a way to create something new from an experience you would never have chosen for yourself.

Don't jump to positivity before you've had the chance to feel the impact of your setback. Allow yourself to fully feel the upset and express your emotions. Go cry in the bath if you have to. Find support if you need it or take time to yourself if that's what works for you. This is your journey and only you know what brings you comfort. And only you know how long that grieving period needs to take.

When you've had a chance to feel your feelings, then you can bring mindfulness into play. Putting a positive spin on a churning sea of emotion is a disaster waiting to happen. Real healing comes when you face your pain and your fear. When you've let it play out, you'll have a chance to regroup.

Sadly, life doesn't stop throwing things at you when you have breast cancer. As well as dealing with your illness, you may have to cope with death in the family, financial issues or a relationship breakup. Sometimes it will feel like it will never stop raining on you. Weirdly, those may be the times when you start to find it funny. There can be a point when the bad news is so ridiculous you can't help but laugh because it's impossible to imagine it getting any worse.

The prescription is always the same, even for setbacks. Feel it, take care of yourself, seek support and prioritize. There's only so much you can cope with, so be realistic about what you can handle and get help.

Whatever your setback, try to stay in the present moment. It doesn't help to second-guess your past choices. Stay in the now and look at how you can best move forward. It may mean learning to accept a choice that you've previously rejected. If that's the case, stay away from thoughts of regret. If it had been the right choice at that time, you'd have done it. Now that things have changed, you need an open mind to review all options. Remind yourself how much you've come through already. It will give you the strength to go on. You're being tempered by the fire and will emerge as strong as steel.

Now that you have body, emotions and mind all attuned to healing, let's move on to finding meaning and purpose in your breast cancer journey.

Clarity of mind checklist ✓

- Be mindful and stay in the present moment

- Feel gratitude to shift your mindset

- Make choices from a clear and calm state

- Notice repetitive negative thought patterns

- Choose thoughts that uplift you

- Self-soothe when you feel overwhelmed

- Journal daily to express concerns and clear your mind

- Create an Aliveness Oracle to bring light to dark days

- Have a compelling vision to pull you through

- Learn to be resilient in the face of setbacks

CHAPTER 7

Soulfulness

Making change meaningful and finding purpose

'If people would get in touch with their spirits, they would be able to heal, emotionally and physically.'

ELISABETH KÜBLER-ROSS

The most striking awareness that breast cancer brought me was how disconnected I was from my body, my desires and my sense of self as a woman. I had managed to grow a tumour the size of a grapefruit – it was eventually found to be 13cm – without even noticing it was there. And then there was my purpose. When life was looking like it might be short in supply, I was forced to examine what I was doing with whatever time I had left.

Like most people who've gone through a difficult time in the past, I was so often waiting for the other shoe to drop. Long before cancer poked its ugly head around the door, long periods of chronic illness and a bad breakup had left me expecting that disaster was just around the corner, so I buried myself in my work and kept my expectations at survival level.

I took on work that I really didn't want to do, just because I was terrified of refusing it in case nothing else showed up. While I was fascinated by meaning and purpose, I had a huge blind spot about how it was missing in my own life.

The knight on the white charger that rode in to save me was breast cancer. It brought its own dark gifts, the kind that appear foul but secretly are the fairest of them all. It holds up a mirror to your life and asks you to choose what's important.

To understand the transformative power of your illness, you need to see it as an archetypal journey. The mythologist Joseph Campbell discovered that societies around the world have always told the same story of a hero's journey, a mono-myth with infinite variations in the telling. It's the story of our lives, as we leave our ordinary world by a willing or unwilling call to adventure, endure ordeals and tests in another world, and return to the ordinary world anew, bearing the gifts of our journey.

Breast cancer takes you to that other world. The rules have changed. Nothing is the same. You're living a new normal, constantly confronted by trials and ordeals. In this new world, all that is not essential is stripped away. Perhaps for the first time, even in the midst of it all, we can see clearly what is of value.

This is where the rubber hits the road. If you believe your life has purpose, this is where you'll find it. That's the paradox of illness – it pushes us to our limits, far beyond what we think we can endure, and yet it shows us who we truly are. At a time when we feel divorced from all that we've held dear, and life feels like it's hanging in the balance, we come home to ourselves.

The territory of the soul

'And every day, the world will drag you by the hand,
yelling "This is important! And this is important!
And this is important! You need to worry about
this! And this! And this!" And each day it's up
to you, to yank your hand back, put it on your
heart and say, "This is what's important."'

IAIN S. THOMAS, THE GRAND DISTRACTION[1]

In Chapter 4: Embodiment you learned to nourish and embrace your body, even in the most difficult of circumstances. In Emotional Ease you explored the patterns and traumas that have held you back, and learned to calm the waves of feeling. In Clarity of Mind, you developed the discernment to observe your thoughts and develop mental resilience. Now we're in the territory of the soul.

Everything you've experienced until this moment is leading to a life where you return from your journey with the treasure. We're going to look at how to take all you've learned about yourself and go forward to create a life of purpose and meaning.

When we've spent our lives without nourishing ourselves – adapting to people and circumstances – we may not even know what it is that we want. Breast cancer offers an invitation to discover what's most fulfilling for you. The answers may be buried in the past, they may be long-cherished dreams or something new may evolve from all you've experienced.

As you become more connected to your true self and your own needs, a sense of purpose will emerge and you'll know that you're on the right path. Only self-enquiry and self-knowledge can take you there. No-one else can do it for you. This is how illness transforms – it strips away everything so you can begin anew, with a clear sense of what's important.

Remember that scene in the movie *Runaway Bride* where Richard Gere forces Julia Roberts to sit down to breakfast and choose the type of eggs she likes? She doesn't know, because she's always had whatever her boyfriend had – scrambled, poached or fried – but she has no idea which one she prefers. On the way to understanding what we want, every authentic choice reinforces our sense of meaning and purpose. Even how we like our eggs.

~ THE POWER OF THREE ~

Whenever you're struggling to find what's important to you, use the power of three to focus in on what matters to you.

1. Look around you. What are your three favourite things in your home? Ask yourself why you love them and what they represent to you.

2. Think of three famous people who inspire you – what qualities do they express that you admire?

3. Ask yourself which three songs you most love and why? What do the lyrics say to you?

Now start to get a picture of what these people and things have in common. Is it a quality or feeling, or is it an aspiration? At this point you're not trying to nail down a purpose. You're simply exploring the values that are important to you and how you want to feel. Keep exploring the threes. Try thinking of your favourite holiday destinations, artworks or films. Every answer will bring you closer to what you truly desire.

~

Whole woman review

To deepen your experience of authenticity and purpose, we're going to go in search of the lost dreams of childhood, the passions you haven't pursued and what's beginning to fascinate you now. We'll take a sweeping view of all the aspects of your life, to help you build the habits and routines that will support you in living life your way.

And we'll explore the final step of the hero's journey – the return to the world with a treasure that has the power to transform others as the hero herself has been transformed. You'll find the treasure unique to you in the dark gift of your personal breast cancer experience.

Let's start with a quick audit of where you are with the elements we've covered in earlier chapters. Jot a few notes now, just to keep you on track. This is a gentle enquiry, to start noticing what works for you. Don't use this review as an opportunity to beat yourself up. Celebrate the progress you've made and it will give you the impetus to make more changes.

Body

How's your diet? Are you doing any regular exercise? Have you treated yourself to supportive therapies like acupuncture or massage? Are you listening more to how your body feels?

What I've changed:

....

....

....

What I'd like to change:

....

....

....

Emotions

How are you feeling, emotionally? Have you found the right people to support you? Are you able to ask for help? Are you being gentle with yourself and allowing yourself to express your emotions? Are you setting firmer boundaries with people?

What I've changed:

....

....

....

What I'd like to change:

....

....

....

Mind

Are you staying in the present moment more? Can you rein your mind back in when it starts to wander into worst-case scenarios? Are you treating yourself more kindly? Are you speaking up for yourself? Are you making decisions more confidently?

What I've changed:

....

....

....

What I'd like to change:

....

....

....

Creating balance

Also ask yourself where are you most at home – in the realm of the body, the emotions, the mind or the soul? That will give you more clues about how to restore balance. Some of us do a lot of physical activity but ignore the spiritual. Others stay in the realm of the mind, safe from troubling emotions. Some are content to focus all their attention on the mental and spiritual, but remain disconnected from their body and emotions.

What are your areas of comfort and which ones do you avoid? Write a little about what you've discovered.

....

....

....

Everything we're doing is focused on self-care and the ultimate expression of self-care is to be compassionate with yourself. Some days you'll feel stronger than others. It goes with the territory. Accept yourself no matter what. Be your own greatest support. Be forgiving and kind to yourself and watch how your life will change.

As you bring all these elements of your life into balance, you can more easily attune to what it means to be living your life on purpose. When you're being pulled in every direction by other people's demands and the chaos of life, it's impossible to hear your own inner voice. Only when you take control of your time and your energy can you really feel what has value for you and act on it. Only then can you be guided by your own heart.

To find purpose, you must find meaning. And meaning isn't universal, it's personal. Your life, your journey and your dance with cancer – it's all unique to you. The meaning you draw from it will be too.

The message in the madness

What if this illness had a message for you? What if it had a purpose, and it was happening *for* you, not *to* you? If you knew it had a message for you, what do you think it would be?

Stop for a moment now, sit quietly, breathe deeply and ask your breast cancer that question – *What are you here to tell me?* Listen for an answer and then jot it down here. It could be a word or a sentence. You're just listening for a glimmer of an idea. Don't expect it to arrive fully formed. You may be lucky and it could come through clearly, or it may take time to percolate. Write down whatever comes to you now and allow the idea to develop over time.

....

....

....

If you're struggling with this process, here's a quick mental bypass to get you out of overthinking and into your inspired mind. Say to yourself, 'I don't know what my breast cancer is here to tell me, but if I did, it would be ...'.

This little trick allows your creative mind to come into play. You may feel as if you're making it up, but go with whatever comes up for you. Listen to what pops into your mind without judgement. Later on, you can look at how true it is for you, but for the moment, simply be receptive.

Take what you've heard into your daily life. Start noticing what's joyful for you and what feels joyless. Notice any of the behaviours that this message has highlighted. Be a detective in your own life, identifying when you're doing things out of obligation and when you're doing things that make your soul sing.

Your natural rhythms

The voice of the soul is a quiet one. It needs a slower pace and an ear attuned to your inner world, not the outer one. Pay attention to how you feel at different times of the day, to get a sense of your natural rhythms. Are you a morning, afternoon, evening or night person? When do you come into your own? When you work with your natural rhythms, you're more attuned to your purpose and life feels easier.

Let what you learn about yourself help you to restructure your life so it works for you, not against you. Our routines can help or hinder us. Are you throwing yourself into the day too quickly, when naturally you prefer a slower start? Or are you working too late when you've long lost the energy to carry on? Notice when your energy is high and when it sags. When you know what your body wants, you can start to build your life and routines around it.

Although I wake early, I really don't have a lot of concentration until later in the day. I prefer a gentle start with meditation and Morning Pages. Then I do everything that requires a shorter attention span – like emails and social media – before lunch. Anything that needs deeper concentration and creative thought gets done in the afternoon or evening.

I work from home, so I'm in control of my schedule, but even if you go out to work you can try to organize your workflow to suit your rhythms. The same applies to socializing. If you skew towards the introverted side of the scale, you'll want more time to yourself. If you're more extroverted, you'll enjoy having company more often. The key is to be in touch with what you need.

As you settle into a better rhythm in your life, you'll be more attuned to what's working for you. Purpose is found in the small things. We tend to expect that purpose will arrive with a fiery passion, but more often it's a gentle flame that needs nurturing.

Let's look at a few different areas of your life – past and present – to see where your gifts of meaning and purpose may be hiding.

Finding your gifts

What were your childhood dreams? Consider the careers you imagined, places you wanted to live, things you wanted to do – and ask yourself how much your current life has in common with those dreams. You're looking for themes more than precise matches.

....

....

....

What was important to you as a child? Was it freedom, making a difference or travelling the world? Did you want to win an Oscar, break a sports record, or top the music charts? How did you want to be seen? Jot down the main themes, and whether any of them are finding expression in your life at the moment.

....

....

....

How did you play when you were a child? Did you like to paint or make things? Did you create songs, stories or plays? Were you into team activities like sports? What was fun for you then? What place does fun have in your life now? Make a note of what you discovered about your childhood sense of fun and expression and how you experience that now.

....

....

....

What has always come easily to you? Are you a good listener? Do you have musical or writing talent? Are you the peacemaker or a trouble-shooter? Are you a born leader? The talents that are most natural to us are usually the ones we undervalue. Because we can do them easily, we assume others are the same.

Think back to your childhood talents, what you offer in your relationships now and the skills that you rely on as second nature at work. Write down what your natural talents are and how you're expressing them in your life now.

....

....

....

Expressing your values

Having taken inspiration from the past, we can explore some other aspects of your life as it is now. We're trying to get a sense of where you're spending your time and attention to relax or entertain yourself. You may not have realized how your interests can point to a theme that runs throughout your life.

One of the things I adore is perfume. Curiously, I had no idea how important that was to me until I took my first course in making fragrance. I suddenly realized that I had an enormous wardrobe of scents dating back decades, because every time I went on a business trip, I would use the time waiting for planes to seek out new perfumes. It was an unconscious habit that eventually turned into a creative pursuit that became enormously fulfilling for me.

Look for clues in your own life from the things that you've collected or found fascinating to read about, or the hobbies that you've always thought you'd like to pursue one day.

What do you like to do culturally? This can be art, music, sport, food or any kind of cultural event or activity. What is it about this that feels fulfilling to you? Make a note of where your interests lie and why they fascinate you.

....

....

....

What social issues are you concerned about? How do you feel about animal rights, feminism, human trafficking, aged care, poverty, endangered species, accessible education or protecting the environment? Write down the ones that fire you up or make you feel sad. You're trying to get to your passions here – to understand what lights you up and calls you to make a difference.

....

....

....

How do you express creativity in your life? Are you a problem-solver? Do you make things, write, sing or bake? Do you have a strong style in décor or fashion? Are you always the one people come to for ideas? Creativity comes in all shapes and sizes. You may be dismissing your own creative activities because you're not pursuing them on a large scale, but they have enormous value in your life as they allow you to express your own unique vision. Explore how creativity runs through your life now and envision how it could become an even bigger part of your life going forward. Write down what you discover.

....

....

....

What do you crave? What's missing from your life? Is it time with an old friend, solitude, deep conversation, a massage, a day by the ocean or a night out on the town? What would you absolutely love to do, but haven't done for a very long time or maybe never? Write down your dreams, the ways you'd love to indulge yourself, and the things you love doing that you never seem to find time for.

....

....

....

What brings you the deepest joy? What are you doing when you feel you're truly yourself and passionate about life? It could be something creative, an outdoor activity, appreciating beauty in art or design, running, spending time with your family or your partner, writing or volunteering. It doesn't have to be something big – it could be a small moment of connecting to nature or sharing what you've learned. What's important is that it makes you feel alive and utterly yourself. Make a note of the activities and aspirations that set your heart on fire.

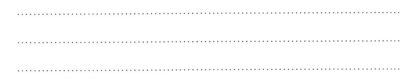

....

....

....

Looking back at all that you've learned from these questions, choose three activities that would bring you joy or give your life meaning and commit to doing them this week. Jot them down here, then make a date in your diary to set aside a specific time when you're going to do them. Taking action brings your dreams closer.

....

....

....

Living the questions

Breast cancer invites you to discover how well you've learned to nourish yourself, and to resolve to live authentically for the rest of your life. That is something only you can teach yourself. Start living each day with the questions that take you closer to who you really are and how you want to live.

Pay attention to your answers to these questions, and live each day asking yourself what's important to you and what it is that you love to do. A new purpose will arise from that. Your illness has brought a huge potential for growth and rebirth. Don't miss that opportunity.

While the path of self-discovery is exciting and rewarding, it doesn't come without pain. As you delve into old memories and long-lost passions, there may be regret and sorrow. To truly release the past and find the gifts that have been lost to us, we cannot avoid pain. When it comes, accept it and allow it. It will pass. Don't let it discourage you. As

Joseph Campbell says, 'The cave you fear to enter holds the greatest treasure.' We live our lives trying to avoid sorrow, yet we're carrying it within us and it's a heavy weight.

There is an enormous relief and freedom that comes from facing the ghosts of the past, dealing with disappointments and confronting our beliefs about ourselves that arose from what happened to us. Your journey with breast cancer gives you the chance to rebuild your life and begin again. The house has been washed away – don't rebuild it on sand. Set your foundations firmly in the bedrock of self-knowledge, self-acceptance and self-care.

Be an active participant in your healing and the new life that springs from it. Old patterns may rear up, because changing deep-seated ways of being takes time, but you're on a new road. You're only looking back so you'll know better where you're headed. Grasp this chance with both hands. Your life depends on it.

Spiritual practice

One of the fastest ways to attune to your inner voice and stay on track is to develop a daily spiritual practice. And by spiritual, I don't necessarily mean religious. We're talking about a personal practice that's aligned with your beliefs and makes you feel supported and purposeful. If you already follow a faith, then use your daily practice to reinforce that.

For those who have no particular religion, but do have a sense of spirituality, daily practice will help you to feel calm and centred. It will also bring a greater depth of meaning to your life. And if you've always thought that stuff is a bit too woo-woo for you, bear with me. Give it a whirl and you'll see the benefits.

Journaling for purpose and guidance

We've talked about journaling before – doing a Morning Page as a brain dump and to clear your mind. Another way to use it is as a direct line to your inner guidance. Each morning, after you've done your Morning Page, sit quietly for a few moments and formulate a question you'd like an answer to. It doesn't have to be a huge one – it's probably best not to start with something you're really worried about – and just let what comes to mind flow out onto the page.

You can call this inspired writing or daily guidance, but the purpose is the same – to tap into your intuition so you can live your life more authentically and soulfully. Here are a few questions you might want to try to get you started.

- What would you have me receive?

- What would you have me know?

- What do I need to let go of?

- What do I need to embrace?

- Who do I need to forgive?

- What does my body want?

- What's my next step in restoring wellness?

You can add a single page of guidance and inspiration to your morning routine, to set you up for the day in a positive and purposeful way. A regular practice becomes an anchor in your life, something that always returns you to a state of peace.

The more you do the same activity on a regular basis, the more your mind and body will become accustomed to it and automatically enter a state of relaxation as you begin. It helps to do it in the same place and at roughly the same time each day. When you have a consistent practice, the benefits build on each other so you naturally become more focused and attuned to your inner world.

In spiritual practice you're calling upon the life force within you to support you in restoring your wholeness. For some that's God, while for others it's the Universe, Source or the angels. If you have no strong beliefs you could just call on life itself to inspire you. Whatever your faith, you're drawing upon a source of support that comes from your inner world, that can put you back in touch with who you truly are, rather than who you are in response to others' needs. When the world outside is incredibly challenging, tapping into your inner world can offer a wellspring of comfort, inspiration, guidance and joy.

Spiritual practice can help you restore a sense of your own beauty and worth too, when it's been challenged by disfigurement or the energy-draining side-effects of cancer treatment. You can learn to look softly upon yourself, and receive your own compassion and care.

A two-way heart

Treating yourself gently, you can begin to develop a heart that is capable of receiving, not just giving. With a two-way heart, you'll be participating in the world in a way that is loving to yourself as well as to others.

~ RECEIVING LOVE ~

Here's a quick exercise you can use at any time of day – in the morning to set you up for a peaceful day, during the day when you feel like you've lost your centre and in the evening before bed so you can drift off to sleep comforted by your own self-care.

1. Sit quietly for a moment and put your hand on your heart. Feel it pulsing beneath your fingers and say silently to yourself, 'I receive my own love.'

2. Repeat this phrase until you feel your heart is full and you're comforted and at peace.

~

If you want to take this a little further, you can do a quick mini-meditation on allowing your heart to give and receive.

~ THE TWO-WAY HEART MEDITATION ~

Relax and breathe deeply, placing your hand on your heart, and practise receiving your own love as you've just learned. Then follow these steps to develop a gentle rhythm of receiving and giving love.

1. When you feel comfortable receiving your own love, and your heart feels full, send love out to someone or something you care for. It could be a person, an animal or nature. Feel that love flowing out to them as your heart pulses beneath your hand.

2. Now allow that love to flow back to you, back into your heart and receive it fully. Let a steady rhythm begin – sending love outwards as you breathe out, and receiving love as you breathe in.

3. Continue receiving and giving love for a couple of minutes until you feel complete with the process.

~

Breast cancer will challenge all of your beliefs on how lovable you are, until finally you become the one who defines it for yourself. You can learn to love yourself and your body in a way that honours all that you have been through. Your scars are reminders of hard-won wisdom and have their own dark beauty.

In Japan there's an art called *kintsukuroi*. It creates beauty in damaged ceramics by repairing the cracks with gold, so the broken places not only look more beautiful, but have more value. It's a way of celebrating breakage and repair as a natural cycle of life that creates a new beauty, not something to be ashamed of or hidden. When breast cancer makes you feel lost and unlovable, remember that you're becoming more beautiful, more valuable and stronger than before in all those broken places.

Building a gratitude bank

Gratitude is another powerful approach to have in your spiritual toolkit. It puts you in touch with what's important to you, and brings a sense of hopefulness to days that are dark. Even in the most challenging of times, there's always the smallest glimmer of light. It could be as simple as you're still here for another day, for once you slept through the night or a kind friend cheered you up with a phone call. Build your gratitude bank every day to give you the strength to stay hopeful, come what may.

A gratitude journal is a great place to start for getting into the gratitude habit. Integrate it into your morning practice by listing three things you're grateful for, or note down the moments that made your heart sing each night before you go to bed. You can just stop and smell the roses, taking time to notice what inspires gratitude throughout the day, but the act of writing makes it more concrete. If you have a journal, then you'll also have something to go back to in tough moments – a permanent little source of joy to make you smile again.

Now that we've explored how to restore balance in your body, your emotions, your mind and your spirit, let's move out of treatment mode to look at life beyond breast cancer.

Soulfulness checklist ✓

- See your illness as a transformative journey

- Review what you've changed and what still needs to change

- Assess where you're out of balance – body, emotions, mind or spirit

- Be compassionate with yourself

- Ask your illness what message it has for you

- Discover your natural rhythms

- Find and honour your unique gifts

- Define what's important to you in life

- Create a regular spiritual practice

- Learn to receive love fully

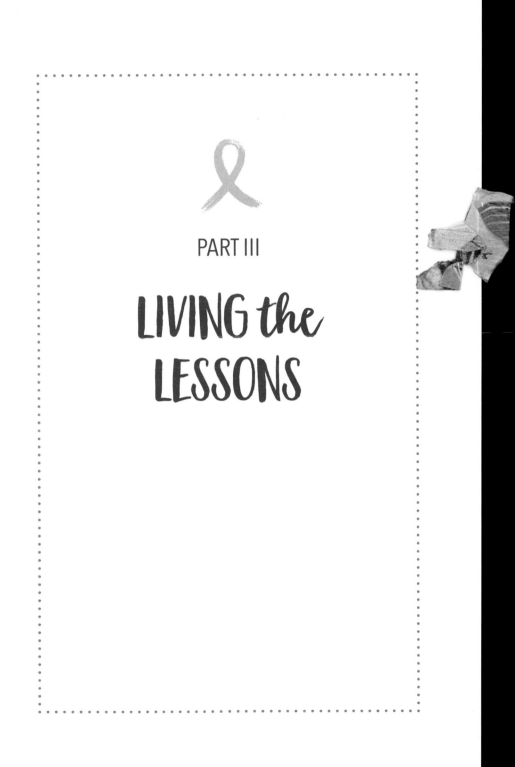

PART III

LIVING the LESSONS

CHAPTER 8

Lotus in Bloom

Reconstruction and life after cancer

*'My mission in life is not merely to survive, but
to thrive, and to do so with some passion, some
compassion, some humor, and some style.'*

MAYA ANGELOU

Breast cancer is a hard thing to put behind you. The scars remain and the results of cancer treatment are so variable that you can live in constant fear of recurrence. While reconstruction can rebuild the resemblance of a breast, it will never be the same.

Some women are lucky enough to have immediate reconstruction, while others, like me, may have to wait years for theirs, living with a single breast as a daily reminder of the disease. It's challenging to try to move out of the cancer patient mindset when the evidence of it is all around you.

For me, reconstruction has brought the freedom to forget about breast cancer. To be able to get up in the morning and throw on some clothes without having to worry about disguising a mastectomy is an enormous relief. It may seem like a small and superficial thing, but it's the ability to forget – even for a moment – that is so powerful.

Not all women will opt for reconstruction and many will not need to. If cancer surgery is a successful lumpectomy, their surgical journey is over. But those of us who have had mastectomies will need to decide if we stop there or go on to have reconstruction and the additional work of reconstructing a nipple.

> ## Mastectomy tattoos
>
> *If reconstruction isn't right for you, you may want to consider a tattoo to cover your mastectomy scar. Mastectomy tattoos are rapidly becoming an art form that helps breast cancer survivors to create something beautiful from their scars.*
>
> *The US charity P.ink connects survivors with tattoo artists who can bring their vision of a healing mastectomy tattoo to life, and it funds tattoos in North America. They also recommend mastectomy tattoo specialists around the world. See www.p-ink.org for recommended artists and inspiration for your tattoo.*

Reconstructive surgery

There are three main types of reconstructive surgery – with implants, using your own body tissue or a combination of both. You may have a couple of options to choose from, depending on your breast size. Your body shape and composition will also affect which types of surgery will work for you.

In my case, the technique of moving muscle and tissue from my back to create a new breast wasn't an option, as I didn't have sufficient tissue there for it to be workable. Your surgeon can advise you on the procedures that will be appropriate options for your body and your breast size. Then you need to consider the risks of each, your preference for having implants or using your own tissue and whether a shorter or lengthier recovery period best suits you. Make sure you've seen what the results look like before you undertake any kind of reconstruction. Your breast cancer nurse or surgeon should have a selection of images to show you, or may even refer you to a support group where you can speak to women who've had the procedure.

My reconstructive surgeon insisted I attend a local group before committing to surgery, which was invaluable. I had the chance to see different types of reconstruction and what the scarring would look like some years later, as well as listening to women's individual stories of how long it took them to recover. There was also a short presentation by a surgeon, giving us details of the procedure and the initial recovery period, so we would know what to expect at every stage of our hospital stay. If this isn't on offer where you are, at least ask your surgeon to put you in touch with a previous patient, so you can get a better idea of what to expect and how long recovery really takes.

Implants

Implant surgery is less invasive than reconstruction with your own tissue, but it does come with its own issues. The implants won't last forever and you'll probably need an additional surgery to replace them in around 10 years. Implants also stay cool, and don't feel as soft or warm as a breast reconstructed from your own tissue. It's harder to achieve a more natural shape if only one breast is being reconstructed with an implant, and both breasts will age differently too. An implanted breast will not sag with age like a natural breast and could end up looking higher than the other one.

If you're having an immediate reconstruction you're most likely to be offered implant reconstruction. It's a shorter surgery, with a faster recovery time than other reconstructive options. Implants have an outer shell made from silicone elastomer and are filled with silicone gel or saline. Silicone gel is used for most reconstructive implants as it tends to give a more natural look and is less heavy than saline.

If you're considering implant surgery, do investigate the complications that can arise with implants, which can include capsular contracture, which is a response of the body's immune system to a foreign material. Internal scar tissue forms a capsule around the implant, tightening and compressing it, causing the breast to harden and become misshapen and painful. Additionally, implants can rupture and leak their contents into your body. Before you decide on implant surgery, make sure to consult your surgeon on potential side effects and do your own research on the type of implant being proposed to you.

If you're having an implant reconstruction, you could be in hospital for up to three days and recovery time is around four to six weeks, depending on whether your reconstruction takes place at the same time as your mastectomy.

Reconstruction using your own tissue

There are two main types of reconstruction using your own tissue. A pedicled flap is where the tissue remains attached to its blood vessels at one end, so it's not necessary to cut the blood supply to the muscle. In a free flap, the section of tissue is removed completely, along with its blood vessels, and microsurgery is used to reattach it to create a reconstructed breast. A free flap is more complicated and requires a much longer surgery and recovery time.

Here are a few of the most common types of own-tissue reconstructive surgery, although there are several more, which can include removing tissue from your bottom or thighs.

Pedicled flap

One of the most popular pedicled flaps uses the latissimus dorsi (LD) muscle just beneath your shoulder blade to move tissue from your back to create a new breast. Some of the flap's skin forms the new breast shape, while the muscle and fat fill out the volume. If the new breast isn't large enough to match the other natural breast, then an implant may also be used to add volume. You could be in hospital for anything from four days to a week for this type of surgery, and the recovery time is around four weeks.

DIEP flap

This is a free flap procedure that takes skin and fat – but no muscle – from your lower abdomen to reconstruct a breast.

While it's a more natural option, there's significant scarring involved, not only to the breast but also across the stomach above the bikini line. It's called DIEP because it uses deep blood vessels called inferior epigastric perforators.

The recovery time is significant as it's a lengthy operation, and you'll need to be in good health to undergo it. It comes with its own risks, including the chance that if there isn't a good blood supply to the tissue it may die and the reconstruction will fail. Again, consult your surgeon to understand all the possible risks and outcomes, and do your own research as well. You'll be in hospital for around seven days with this type of surgery and the recovery period is several months.

I had this type of reconstruction and it has been a wholly positive experience for me. I was blessed with an extremely precise and talented surgeon with an excellent support team, in whom I had the utmost confidence. Don't settle for anything less. The operation is long and complex, with a lengthy recovery period. Before you commit, you should be satisfied that you're in the right hands and that this is the right choice for you. On the upside, as a large chunk of your stomach will be removed to create your new breast, you'll effectively get a tummy tuck – and a new belly button – into the bargain.

SIEA flap

The super inferior epigastric artery (SIEA) flap uses skin and fat from the lower abdomen like the DIEP flap, but it uses superficial rather than deep blood vessels. Whether this technique can be used depends on whether you have SIEA blood vessels or adequate vessel size, and the majority of women do not. The hospital stay and recovery period is similar to the DIEP flap, and likely shorter.

TRAM flap

This uses your large tummy muscle – the rectus abdominis muscle – and removes skin transversely, hence the name. TRAM procedures can be pedicled or free flaps. TRAM reconstructions are common because the tissue used is similar to breast tissue, but due to the severing of muscle they can result in a weakening of the abdominal wall.

Both the pedicled and free flap TRAM reconstructions run the risk of tissue death. Pedicled TRAM flaps may have insufficient blood circulation, and while free TRAM flaps also carry some of that risk, it's less common. It's important to discuss all available options with your surgeon, to ensure you choose the reconstructive technique that best suits your body and has a level of risk that you can live with. TRAM flap surgeries usually involve a hospital stay of around five days, with a recovery period of approximately six weeks.

If you have large breasts, whichever reconstructive route you take, you may need to have the other breast reduced to match. Depending on your surgeon, this will be done at the same time or in a separate operation. If you're having a large operation like a DIEP flap with a long recovery period, think carefully about having two separate operations. Anaesthesia carries its own risks and multiple surgeries take their toll on your body. If you can find a surgeon who is willing to reconstruct and do a reduction at the same time, you'll not only feel better about having both breasts returned to a more natural balance in a single operation, but you'll also be saving yourself waiting time between surgeries and recovery time.

Nipple reconstruction

When you've had your reconstruction, you can consider whether or not to pursue nipple reconstruction. It's usually offered to you around four to six months after your reconstruction, when the swelling has subsided so the nipple can be positioned accurately.

You could opt for a flat nipple tattoo, have a flap created from your reconstructed breast tissue to give the raised look of a nipple – with tattooing to colour the flap – or have the nipple-sharing graft where part of your remaining nipple is grafted to your reconstructed breast to create smaller nipples of the same colour and texture.

Recovery time

While I've given some rough recovery times here for guidance, it really is a very personal thing. I tend to bounce back quickly – often overestimating just how well I am – only to discover later that I've taken on too much too soon.

Be gentle with yourself and allow as much time as possible for recovery. You'll be more tired than you

> *expect, in pain and discomfort for some time, and*
> *have all sorts of odd little aches for months afterwards.*
> *Pay close attention to how your body feels and don't*
> *overcommit yourself.*

A word on expectations

Managing your expectations when it comes to reconstruction will make the process easier. Whatever you choose, a reconstructed breast isn't ever going to be just like your original breast. That ship has sailed. What you'll have is a breast mound, a nipple – or not, depending on your choice – and quite a bit of scarring. The size is going to depend on what can be achieved with your tissue and it may not heal as quickly as you'd like. When you can accept that it's going to be different, you can love it for what it is. Go into the process with realistic expectations and you'll be much happier with the results.

A post-cancer mindset

With your reconstruction complete, you can begin to look at life after breast cancer. This means coming to terms with your experience and realizing that while it's not easy to put it behind you, it has shaped your life. Your job now is to shift your identity from cancer patient to cancer survivor.

What most people don't realize about cancer is that the threat never really goes away. You have to learn to live with it. You can cut it out, but circulating cancer cells mean it may reappear elsewhere in your body. You may be cancer-free for a long period, but it could recur. That's a lot of uncertainty to deal with. Any of those things may happen. And they may not. The only way you're going to have peace of mind is if you decide that you've done all you can – assuming you've taken all the physical, emotional, mental and spiritual steps to return your body to balance – and that you're going to get on with your life.

I don't say that lightly. I'm a few years out from my original diagnosis now, and yet occasional fears of recurrence still arise. They probably always will. Even with everything I've done on every possible level, I can't say, hand on heart, that I'll never experience cancer again. However, had I gone down the most traditional of routes there still would have been no guarantee that it wouldn't come back either.

Uncertainty is the territory of cancer. You learn to live with it or you drive yourself mad with worry. Your task now is to stop saying 'I have cancer', and start looking at it as something you used to have. It may seem like a small shift, but it's a huge change in perspective. When you have cancer, you're always waiting for the other shoe to drop, for something unexpected to occur, for the worst to happen. You live in a cycle of dread, fearing the future.

Now it's time to reclaim the future as a positive place. Consider yourself not just a survivor – you're now a thriver. Personally, I don't like using the term 'survivor'. I didn't go through all of this just to survive. I'm toying with the idea of being a cancer 'graduate'. That at least honours the depth of the journey and the lessons learned along the way.

Moving into a post-cancer phase is a shift from healing to wellness. You're out of the woods, and stepping into the light. There's infinite possibility here – a rare opportunity to reboot and begin again with focus and purpose, knowing how precious time really is.

You may find yourself changing your work, your relationships and where you live. That doesn't necessarily mean out with the old and in with the new, but now you have an opportunity to deepen your relationships and spend time doing what is meaningful for you, in ways that bring you joy.

Kissing breast cancer goodbye

Cancer can linger as a constant presence in our lives. As well as using mindfulness to help us move into life beyond breast cancer, we can also remove the associations we have with it. Try some of these ways to cut the cord. You're ready for a new life.

- *Give it a ritual ending – burn your soft prosthesis.*

- *If you used a fragrance to uplift you during treatment, find a new one.*

- *Give yourself a makeover.*

- *Redecorate your bedroom or wherever you spent time recuperating.*

- *Donate your cancer books to charity.*

- *Get rid of anything that reminds you of being ill – even a favourite jumper.*

Making the transition

It may take some time for it to really sink in that your dance with cancer is over. It's been your main focus for so long, it can feel strange to be getting on with life without cancer at the centre of it. The end of treatment can feel abrupt – where something was actively being done, now nothing's happening, and where there was support, suddenly now there's none.

A recent study by Breast Cancer Care[1] in the UK revealed that more than a quarter of women found that the end of hospital treatment was harder than having a breast removed or undergoing chemotherapy. Only one in 10 women felt positive and ready to move on when discharged from treatment, with more than half struggling with anxiety and nearly a third with depression.

We'll go into a more detailed approach to post-cancer wellbeing in a moment, but for now let's look at how to deal with the transition into life without treatment. The end of treatment is not the end of healing – that's an ongoing process. When your approach is to pursue wellbeing to empower your immune system, you're going to be doing that whether treatment is happening or not.

If you're an active participant in your own health, your focus will shift from firefighting to maintenance mode at the end of treatment. But if you've not been very engaged in your healing, then it may come as a bit of a shock when treatment suddenly ends. It could reawaken all the anxiety of diagnosis and leave you wondering if the treatment has been effective. If this is you, then it's never too late to help yourself and seek support.

Go back through the chapters on Embodiment, Emotional Healing, Clarity Of Mind and Soulfulness and start applying those techniques so they become a regular practice. They're not just for the cancer journey – they're the foundations of a healthy life. Reach out for emotional support if you need it. You may find that friends and family expect you to be over it now that treatment has taken place. That's so far from the truth, it's ludicrous. Breast cancer is a traumatic experience that can have emotional repercussions that last for years.

Don't let anyone tell you how you should feel. Honour what you need. Get the support of a breast cancer counsellor or coach, or join life-affirming social media groups and meet-ups for breast cancer survivors. Find a safe space where you can express and overcome your fears. For ongoing support and to continue the *Stronger Than Before* journey, join me in my private Facebook group, Breast Cancer Survive & Thrive Tribe. You'll find the link on my page at www.facebook.com/alisonporterauthor/.

The Breast Cancer Care study also found that the three toughest issues women face after treatment are fear of recurrence, struggling with fatigue and lack of body confidence. To deal with these, practise the tips and techniques that you've already learned in earlier chapters on body, emotions, mind and soul. Here's a quick refresher for you.

Fear of recurrence

To overcome this issue, you need to be mindful and stay in the present moment. Right now, in this moment, you're safe and well. You don't know if it will come back, but you can't ruin the rest of your very precious life terrorizing yourself with the thought of something that may never happen. Stay in the here and now – that's where you can feel safe. The fears may never entirely go away, but you can decide how much you want to entertain them.

Fatigue

If you're struggling with this, the answer is always going to be shameless self-care. Don't overestimate what you can do. Plan to do less. Then, if you have the energy, do more. Your body may still be recovering from surgery or dealing with the side effects of treatment or medications for some time, so treat it gently. Your concentration won't be what it was. You'll tire more easily. Accept that. Speak up at work if people are piling on more responsibility before you're ready for it. Don't stay silent. You can very easily trip into overwhelm when you've had breast cancer, so be realistic about what you can achieve.

Ask for help at home and at work. Normal service should not be resumed automatically. You've changed. You're dealing with a lot of emotions and fears, and all of that can be very draining. Limit the time you spend with draining people, especially if you're finding it hard having returned to work. Make an effort to surround yourself with those who uplift you. Your energy is a finite resource. Be careful how you spend it.

Body confidence

This issue is always going to be tricky, and it will depend on how you felt about your body beforehand, how much surgery you've had and how realistic your expectations are for reconstruction. It's a complex issue that we've looked at in detail in the chapter on Embodiment, but in essence it's a process that takes time.

You're not going to fall in love with a body scarred by surgery overnight. But whenever you choose to accept your body for what it is and look at it with kind eyes, you're another step closer to coming to peace with it. And remember that scars fade. Time changes them from angry marks to faint lines. You won't look the same, but the scars will gradually become less obvious and some will even disappear.

Being body confident is an inside job. Reconstructive surgery won't do it for you. It'll help, but if you don't have realistic expectations you'll always be unhappy with your body. Paradoxically, breast cancer is an opportunity to learn to love your body more than you've ever done before, despite the scarring. Accept that invitation. Unravel all the ways you've been unloving to your body before this even happened. Don't let your scars stand in the way of life or love.

Post-cancer wellbeing

To keep you on track for a more fulfilling future, let's look again at body, emotions, mind and spirit, but in wellness mode this time.

Your body

Firstly, your diet should have evolved to support your body with high-value nutrition. You may have been super gung-ho with your juicing and eating fresh, nutritious food. That doesn't have to change, but you can dial it back to maintenance mode now. Stick to the same principles of keeping your body in balance and avoiding foods that cause an inflammatory response. But if you need a treat now and then, you can be more relaxed about it. Try to make them healthier ones though, and ensure that sugary treats are rare. It's a slippery slope and your immune system needs all the help you can give it to ensure your body stays healthy.

Keep up your regular maintenance treatments for wellness, like acupuncture or massage. Unless you make them a priority, things that seem like indulgences can easily slip off your radar. Take tinctures like echinacea for immune support and use dry brushing to keep your lymphatic system flowing. If you've had lymph nodes removed and are at risk of lymphoedema, consider getting a rebounder and bouncing on it regularly to support the lymph function.

Make sure exercise is a regular part of your life and do it in a way that's joyful for you. If you don't like the gym, don't go there. Walk, dance, take a Zumba class or do yoga instead – it doesn't matter what you do, so long as you keep moving. If you're feeling stressed and in need of re-centring, book a restorative or yin yoga class. They'll give you a good stretch and calm your mind at the same time.

Continue the good work with reducing your toxic load. Choose organic foods where you can, use non-toxic cleaning products and make sure your make-up and bodycare products are all natural or organic. Your body has clearly shown you that it's been overwhelmed and out of balance, and you've been lucky enough to recover. Don't start creating a new toxic soup for it to swim in.

Your emotions

Emotionally, you have a clean slate for building relationships that honour you, both at home and at work. You've been through the fire, you understand yourself and your worth much better and you don't need to tolerate anyone who doesn't respect that. Vote with your feet. If something's not working for you, and you've tried to communicate the issues without success, then leave. It will wear you down again if you continue to stay in situations that aren't good for you, and that will have a knock-on effect on your health. The feisty part of you that came alive to heal you isn't going anywhere. Keep her close to your heart and have the courage to say enough is enough.

Your newfound emotional fluidity will mean you'll still be shedding tears, but now it's not because you're afraid, it's because life touches you deeply. Go with it. There's nothing like a therapeutic cry when you need one. That sensitivity is what makes you perceptive and open to your own inner world. When you can accept your own emotions, you give other people the permission to do the same. We're all just trying to hold it together in difficult times. Cut yourself some slack and let your emotions flow through you and wash away. Hold them lightly and they won't frighten you.

You'll still be processing some grief from all you've been through. Don't worry that it will overwhelm you or feel guilty for looking back rather than forwards. Those moments will come, you'll feel them, and they'll pass like summer rain. They're not here for the duration, they're just passing through.

Get excited about what's coming up in your life. Make things happen. Do what you've always wanted to do. If not now, when? No more excuses. No more worrying if you're going to be around to see it through. Do it anyway. There are no guarantees for anyone, whether they've had cancer or not. We don't know how long our lives will be. We just need to use and appreciate the time we have.

Love the ones you love more than ever before. Spend time with people who light you up. Make relationships a priority. Meet up with friends more often. Have deeper conversations. Let the ones who supported you in the dark times have the pleasure of your company now you're healed and ready to take on the world. Have fun. It's life-affirming.

Your mind and spirit

Honour your rhythms, and keep pressure and stress at bay. They are hugely destructive and play a big part in knocking your body out of balance. Prioritize sleep and allow your body to restore itself. Take time out when you need it and plan more getaways. Don't let work pressures take their toll. Ask for more resources or adjust your schedule. If an aspect of your work causes intense stress, see if you can outsource it. Beware of taking on too much, shouldering too much responsibility, or saying yes to things you wish you'd said no to. Old habits die hard, but they can die, and new ones of self-care will grow in strength with repetition.

Commit to exploring meaning in your life. Join groups or movements, volunteer, paint your prayers or write the stories that need to be told. Add your voice to issues that are important to you. If you have a talent, share it. If self-confidence is a struggle, it's easier to get out of your own way if you're doing something to benefit others.

Purpose is doing the small things that count every day. It's being aligned with who you are and who you're meant to be. Keep asking yourself if this choice is taking you closer to your dream or further away. That's how you keep yourself accountable and grow great things from small beginnings – with good choices and consistent action. Don't wait for purpose to reveal itself to you before you take action. Keep doing what feels good and right, and delight in where it leads you.

Facing the future with confidence

From all that you've discovered about yourself and your life up to now, how would you answer the following questions?

What is it that I appreciate now more than ever before?

....

....

....

What have I learned from my dance with breast cancer?

....

....

....

How does that make me want to live?

....

....

....

What have I learned that I want to share?

....

....

....

What old dreams or new passions do I want to explore?

....

....

....

What can I no longer tolerate in my life or in the world?

....

....

....

What could I do that would make the rest of my life meaningful?

....

....

....

Breast cancer's darkest gift is the descent into ourselves and all our pain. But what it releases is a capacity to be truly ourselves. Go deep, live large and love yourself. You made it. Now it's time to grow and love and laugh, more fully than ever before.

Life after cancer checklist ✓

- Have reasonable expectations for reconstruction
- Put the identity of cancer patient behind you
- Consider yourself a breast cancer graduate
- Find the support you need at the end of treatment
- Use mindfulness to overcome fears of recurrence
- Treat yourself gently to manage fatigue
- Double down on acceptance and self-love for body issues
- Maintain all your good work on body, emotions, mind and spirit
- Live what you have learned about yourself
- Build a life that's meaningful for you

CHAPTER 9

Conversations for Family and Friends

Supporting a loved one through breast cancer

*'Listening creates a holy silence. When you
listen generously to people, they can hear truth
in themselves, often for the first time.'*

RACHEL NAOMI REMEN

With a few rare exceptions, I was always shocked by how ill-equipped people were to deal with someone who has cancer. If you're not careful, you can spend more time taking care of people who are upset about your cancer than taking care of yourself. Apart from the emotionally incontinent, who cannot set their feelings aside to accommodate yours, there are also the ones who like to force-feed you their opinion on which type of treatment you should have – or argue with you about choices you've already made.

As well-meaning as people may be, they so very often fail in the execution. Of course it's difficult to know what to say and when, but the most important thing is to listen. So few people can do just that. And it's not just friends and family. Some of the most shockingly insensitive encounters I've had have been with medical professionals – doctors, nurses and ultrasound technicians. They may be trained to deal with the disease, but not all are capable of the sensitivity needed to support women going through an emotionally traumatic experience.

The reason we may struggle with knowing what to say is that culturally we are not adept at sitting with pain – our own or anyone else's. Our society is utterly pain-avoidant. We will do anything not to feel the discomfort of our own pain – numbing it with food, alcohol, work or spending sprees – and we're just as uncomfortable when we see it in others. We turn away, rather than turning towards it.

If you genuinely want to support your loved one through breast cancer, you're going to have to live with her distress. You'll need to acknowledge it to be able to offer comfort. You can't pretend it's not there, or minimize it to keep yourself comfortable. Having a positive outlook is very different to trying to gloss over the reality she is experiencing.

It's OK to say 'I'm so sorry this is happening to you' and 'It must be so hard – my heart goes out to you.' That's a world away from the faux-support of 'You'll be fine' or 'You'll beat this for sure.' That's really just avoidance disguised as positivity. Your loved one knows there's no certainty of outcome, and however positive she may seem on the surface, she still can't avoid the fear that comes with a breast cancer diagnosis. Platitudes about it all being OK ring very false when your life is at risk.

Managing your emotions is key to being able to offer real support. If you're the one getting upset all the time about what's happening to your loved one, you're forcing her to take care of you at a time when she needs to take care of herself. She will stop sharing her feelings with you if she feels overwhelmed by yours.

While you must be true to yourself about how you feel, be sensitive to how that's affecting your loved one. You don't have to put a brave face on it all the time, but be aware that she will be struggling with complex emotions and deep-seated fears, so it will feel overwhelming to constantly handle strong emotions from you too. If you're clearly having difficulty coping with the situation, she will start to feel the need to protect you emotionally at a time when she needs all her energy for herself. Try to be honest without flooding her with your feelings, so she can feel your care and concern as truly supportive.

How to be helpful

Everyone experiences breast cancer differently. Everyone deals with emotions in different ways, so there's not a one-size-fits-all approach to supporting someone as they go through it. However, there are some simple truths you need to bear in mind.

You can't fix this

Your job is to listen. You can't make it better, but you can be there for your loved one. That means letting her speak when she needs to and not pressing her if she doesn't. Some people want to talk it out, while others may have a more internalized process. Just let your loved one be who she is, without judgement.

Some days she may want to open up, and some days she won't. Let her talk on her timetable. Be sensitive to how she's responding. Knowing that you can't fix this, don't try. Acknowledge how she's feeling, so she feels heard and understood. That's a huge gift in itself. You aren't expected to do anything, other than just be there. She simply wants the comfort of knowing that you understand.

When you listen, pay attention

In some parts of the treatment process, there may be long delays before the next step. Constantly hearing the question 'Have you heard anything?' when you've already explained the situation again and again is enormously frustrating. It shows that the person asking hasn't cared enough to pay attention. Write it down if you have to, but try to remember what your last conversation was, so you can pick up where you left off, rather than asking the same question again.

Listening deeply is a skill. Be present, not distracted. Give her your time and your full attention. Don't make it hard for her to open up to you. Set aside your feelings when you're with her, so you can be present to what she needs. Don't make the patient more concerned for you than she is for herself.

Do something kind

A breast cancer patient will hear countless people say 'Let me know if I can do anything', but so few will actually do something thoughtful. Bring a meal to her at home, buy her a magazine subscription, or plan a night in with a comedy film. Just be careful with food and drink as gifts for your loved one, as she may be on a special anti-cancer diet. Ask first. She could be gung-ho with a diet or delighted to have a bit of a blowout.

A moment of thoughtfulness can be a real uplift for a cancer patient. Pop a card in the post to let her know you're thinking of her, or organize a spontaneous outing on a day when she's feeling brighter. Always include her in invitations, but be understanding if she's not up to it. Her energy and moods will be in constant flux, so don't expect her to plan ahead or always stick to arrangements. Don't just drop by, as she may be having a low-energy day. Always call or text first.

Keep your opinions to yourself

Making decisions about cancer treatment is a delicate balance of knowing what's right for your beliefs, your body and your circumstances. Those decisions have to be made at a time of huge emotional turmoil. And even when they're made, there's no absolute certainty that they'll work. Questioning her choices when they've already been decided feels like an attack and adds even more uncertainty to the mix. You can offer information beforehand if it's been requested, but once a decision has been made, accept that she's already made her choice. If you can't say something supportive, don't say anything at all.

Distractions are always welcome

Breast cancer can feel like a full-time job. There are endless hospital appointments for blood tests and scans. If you're offering a loved one a lift to the hospital, plan to go somewhere with her afterwards. You can turn a necessary journey into a bit of fun. Don't always feel as if you have to talk about illness. Having a laugh is so therapeutic.

Feeling normal is a rare treat for a breast cancer patient. Do the things you've always loved to do together, but be sensitive to the amount of energy she may have on the day. When you're going through treatment you tire easily, so don't overestimate her capacity. Rather than plan a whole day out, make it a short jaunt that doesn't require a huge amount of travel. Ask if she'd prefer to go out or would feel more comfortable at home.

Don't assume that you know what's best for her – always ask. And think of new things to do. Treatment feels like the same old routine for long periods of time. There's nothing like novelty to spice things up and reignite someone's zest for life.

Be practical

Your loved one will need a lot more help than she's used to. She may be unable to drive for some time after surgery, or find it difficult to lift or carry anything. Offer to do the shopping, cook a meal, or give her a lift to the hospital or clinic. Be the person who comes to appointments and takes notes, because sometimes it's a lot to take in, or be the one who does the research on treatments she's interested in.

Find ways to lighten the burden. Understand that she may feel uncomfortable asking for help. Keep an eye on what she needs and offer to help before she has to ask. Even if she's usually fiercely independent, she may still need assistance too. If she keeps telling you there's nothing that she needs, get creative and anticipate what she might find useful. Bring some soup or a meal that's easy to heat up. Help around the house wherever you can. Offer to organize bill payments or arrange appointments if she's comfortable for you to do that. In recovery from treatment, a breast cancer patient will have little energy and even less concentration, so even small tasks can seem burdensome. Your help could lift a huge weight from her mind.

Honour her femininity

When your breast has been lopped off, or chemo's drained every ounce of energy from you, or radiation has burned and scarred you, it's an enormous challenge to feel feminine. Surround your loved one with beauty and remind her how beautiful she is to you. Bring flowers or sensual bath oils – if she isn't experiencing sensitivity to fragrance – or give her a stylish scarf that will disguise a mastectomy or keep her warm during treatment.

Suggest an outing to look for new make-up or clothes, or plan a spa day so she feels pampered. You'll know what she takes the greatest pleasure in and what makes her feel attractive. If she's recovering well, maybe suggest a fun dance class to help her feel more connected with her body, or take a restorative yoga class together. Remind her that she's beautiful and loved, regardless of what's going on with her body right now.

Gifts for women with breast cancer

- *When times are hard, we seek comfort. Anything with soft textures will be welcome. Cashmere socks, a cosy scarf, or a comfy wrap are ideal.*

- *Flowers and scented products are beautiful, but if your loved one is going through chemo she may be especially sensitive to fragrance. Be sure to check this before you buy.*

- *Light relief is always desperately needed. If you know her sense of humour, find something that will tickle it.*

- *Send a card, even if you're going to see her soon. It's lovely to know someone is thinking of you.*

Relationships and breast cancer

Every relationship to a cancer patient is different – being a husband or partner isn't the same as being a parent, family member or friend. Partners will shoulder the day-to-day struggle of watching their loved one suffer in a way that's more intimate than most. They run the risk of their loving relationship becoming one of care-taking – lost in the round of endless appointments and treatments.

Parents must face the very real fear of losing their child, while other relatives struggle with how illness affects the family dynamics. Friends find it difficult to know how and when to be there for a patient, without intruding on her intimate and family relationships. Breast cancer takes its toll on everyone.

Your suffering is very real, and you must acknowledge it and seek support too. Here's a little advice for you, to help you offer the best love and care you can, while also making sure that you take care of yourself.

Partners

This is going to demand a level of emotional awareness that perhaps you've never experienced before. You're going to watch your partner in pain and that's something you can't change. In your overwhelming desire for her to survive and stay with you, you may have very strong feelings about what she should do.

But this is not your journey. You're a companion on the path, but how the journey unfolds is not for you to say. Your partner may make choices that terrify you. Support them anyway. She may become more forceful or more frail. Love her anyway. Your job is to support her through this – to care for her fiercely and never let her forget how important she is to you.

You may be surprised that a once-confident partner suddenly seems daunted by making phone calls or arranging appointments. Cancer knocks the stuffing out of you, and it's not easy to get up again. It's a much more emotional experience than your partner ever expected, and that's incredibly draining. Try to be sensitive to days when it's all too much for her. The woman you love is still there. She's just trying to hold it together.

Breast cancer treatments are ugly. There's no nice way to say this. If there's surgery, there will be drains and swelling and leakage. Chemo will drain the life force out of her and radiation may burn her skin. Recovery is slow and her body will be tender for months. Be gentle and be aware that physical contact may be painful. Don't shy away from it, though. Ask. She'll let you know what she's comfortable with. Comfort her when she fears she's lost her femininity along with her breast, or when the scarring feels like complete disfigurement. Your reassurance is what she needs most – reflecting love and desire back to her.

Don't go into denial. Sometimes, in our rush to want everything to go back to normal, we pretend it's not really affecting us as much as it is. Notice what's going on with her and be sensitive to that. Anticipate where she may need help, and don't assume she'll shoulder all the responsibilities she normally does. What seems easy one day may feel like a mountain to climb the next. Take each day as it comes. Remind her how she's progressing. Recovery can feel like endless days stretching out ahead of you with no improvement. If you notice a positive change, encourage her to see that.

Notice what's going on with you too. Care-taking can destroy intimacy, so be sensitive to maintaining your relationship outside the world of breast cancer. Keep doing the things you love to do as a couple. Have a date night, get away for a short trip if you can or try a new activity together when she's feeling well enough.

Seek support. Speak honestly to your good friends or find a support group or counsellor. It may not be your journey, but you'll be absorbing and experiencing a lot of the pain. Allow others to pick up the slack when you're feeling overwhelmed. Take a break if it gets too much. Let family and friends help. Don't do this alone. If you wear yourself out, you'll have nothing left to give when she needs you most.

Parents

It's an unimaginable terror to confront the loss of your child. The thing you've dreaded throughout her life may actually come to pass. This is an enormous trauma which, sadly, can have a great impact on how able you are to offer her comfort. The ties between a parent and child are so infused with family dynamics that it can be hard to set aside habitual ways of relating in order to provide the support that's most needed.

You may be overcome with feelings and unable to contain them when you're with your child, or you may go into denial and try to minimize her fears. You may find it nigh on impossible to release the habit of telling her what to do, and argue with her over her treatment decisions. All of these reactions arise from the love you feel for her, but that will not be recognized. Your child will feel attacked or unsupported, or feel that you're incapable of putting your own emotions aside to offer her comfort. She wants to feel your love and your concern in ways that she can receive it, without being pushed or controlled or having her feelings ignored.

Letting her do what she needs to do and being there for her every step of the way is probably the hardest thing you'll ever do. It will take a huge amount of strength to watch her suffering, while setting aside your own desires to embrace her choices. But this is what real love is. It's honouring the wishes of the one you love, whether you agree with them or not.

Find practical ways to support your child, and her partner if she has one. Offer to be the point of contact for the whole family about her treatment and progress, so she's not inundated with enquiries. Be a buffer for her, so she can focus her energy on getting well again, not keeping everyone up to date.

Be sensitive to how public your child wants to be about her illness, and don't share the diagnosis with anyone until you know she is happy for people to be told. If she's a very private person she may not want anyone outside the immediate family to know. Don't be afraid to talk about it with her. As long as you're willing to listen, you'll do OK. Ask about her experience and don't make pronouncements about what you think should happen. Find out what kind of support she needs and give it to her. Offer to attend appointments, do school runs, cook or clean. Never assume you know what's needed. Your child will be particularly sensitive to how she receives support at this time, so if you think you know best, you're probably wrong.

Be careful who you talk to about your child's illness and your own feelings – keep it to a trusted few. Stories travel fast in families, so don't assume that what you've said won't make it to her ears. You may just be venting about how you wish she'd try a different treatment, because that's what you would do, but when it gets back to her from another source it will feel like a personal attack. Seek support for yourself, because this is an incredibly difficult thing to go through, but choose where you find it carefully. Don't be afraid to seek out counselling. It won't just help you, it will help your child. The better you can cope, the better support you'll be to her.

Family

A breast cancer diagnosis affects the whole family. If it's your mother, it will be terribly frightening for you, and you may struggle to come to terms with the reversal of roles where you now need to be the care-taker rather than the one receiving maternal care. If you're young, you may feel emotionally neglected as your mother's husband or partner focuses their entire attention on helping her to get well.

If this is you, talk to a trusted aunt or family friend – someone who's always been there for you. Just having them there may be enough, or you could find a support group to help you deal with your feelings. To support your mother, do small things to help her out, cheer her up on her bad days and never forget to let her know how much you love her.

If you're a sibling, being supportive can be challenging in many ways. As a woman it will bring up your own fears of a breast cancer diagnosis, along with the complex relationship dynamic that sisters can often have. It will demand real strength to set aside whatever has passed between you so you can be there for her now – and to overcome your own beliefs about what's right for her so you can be truly supportive. However your relationship has unfolded in the past, let this be a line in the sand where you let it all go and decide to support her fully, whatever her decisions may be.

As a man, you may feel a bit remote from her experience and feel awkward bringing it up. Take your lead from your sister. If she wants to open up, listen. Don't try to fix it, just tell her you care. And offer to do practical things. She will love that kind of support. You don't have to be the king of emotional fluidity. If that's not you, do what you can. Just make sure she knows that you're there with her for the journey.

Not all families are tight-knit. Even if you're not close, try to find small ways of offering support. A message, a card, some flowers – just a little something to say you're thinking of your family member. It will be so appreciated.

Friends

Beautiful friends, you have such a unique place in our lives. You may know us better than our families ever will, and you probably know what makes us laugh more than anyone. You're the ones we'll call to let it all hang out when we're afraid of burdening our partners or parents with our despair. You're the rocks we cling to when the waves threaten to drown us.

In a way it can be hardest for you. You'll have to watch us suffer, standing on the sidelines as partners and family take precedence. Yet you're the ones who'll witness our darkest moments as we admit feelings to you that we could never burden our lovers, mothers or siblings with. Even as that's happening, we will still want you to play court jester to us, coaxing a smile out of hiding on a dark day. And you're there for the practical things too. You're the rock stars of our lives, shining brightly come what may.

Because you love us so much, you may struggle with our choices too. If you disagree with our approach to treatment, don't say it. We'll feel undermined. We have enough anxiety. Please don't add to it. Throw that energy into being the entertainment committee instead. Find ways to keep us engaged with life, reminding us of who we used to be, and can be again. You're the ones we can be girlie with, to let our hair down and forget cancer for a while. Consider yourselves to be the queens of distraction. Help us to have fun. We need a little lightening up. No-one wants to do cancer 24/7.

And you're so good at listening. We'll probably tell you all the dreadful tales about the insensitive things that other friends, family or colleagues may have said to us. Just listen and maybe even have a bit of a gallows humour laugh about it, but don't judge them. We need to vent, but we also understand that they're struggling too. It can be frustrating and hurtful, but we get that it's usually because they care and don't know any other way to show it. Be a safe place for us to share how we feel in the moment.

We're going to be more sensitive than you've ever known us. We might make a joke about something one day, but if you carry on in the same vein another day, it may well go down like a lead balloon. We can joke about our situation, but it feels awkward when someone else does. Pay attention to how we're reacting. We can be extra-sensitive when we're trying to heal ourselves. Being so vulnerable, it feels like we're living without an extra layer of skin. Everything seems to strike us in the heart. If you notice that there's another friend who can be very opinionated and pushy with us, have a quiet word with them. Help them to see that real support is unconditional.

Do practical things where you can. Ask us what we're dreading doing and find a way to help. Maybe it's coming with us to an appointment, feeding our animals when we're in hospital or just being there when we come home. It could be pouring a glass of wine on a lousy day or popping the cork on some fizz when we get good results. Or simply emailing us silly cat videos to put a smile on our face when we're going through treatment. Sometimes the smallest acts of love are the most touching.

The worst person to ...

If you were a fan of the improvisational TV comedy show *Whose Line Is It Anyway?* you'll remember there was a segment called 'the worst person to ...', where the comedians would riff on the worst person to encounter in a particular scenario. For a little dark humour, here are some of the things that happened to me that would have made epic 'worst person' breast cancer standup comedy routines. Your loved one is likely to face similar circumstances, so hopefully these stories will help you to recognize the signs and head them off before they develop into real-life black comedy moments.

- While I was still in shock and trying to take in the news that only 6mm of cancer had been found during my mastectomy – following a lumpectomy that had failed to produce clear margins – a breast cancer nurse told me disapprovingly that I should be more grateful, as the surgeon had saved my life.

  Having heard the news only moments before, I was struggling to come to terms with losing my entire breast for a wafer-thin 6mm. When I'd arrived for my appointment, the consultant had already scared the living daylights out of me by asking if I wanted someone with me before giving me the results. I thought he was preparing me for another failure. Without allowing me even a few minutes to process it all, that nurse was telling me how to feel. And this was someone who was allegedly trained to deal with breast cancer patients.

- I lost count of the number of people who would argue with me over treatment choices, never once realizing how invasive that was or how far it overstepped the mark. We don't want to hear what you would do, or what your relative did or what you've researched on the internet, unless we ask you. We definitely don't want to feel like we have to justify our choices. Unsolicited advice is the junk mail of the breast cancer world. Keep it to yourself.

- Perhaps the most shocking thing of all is the glee with which people will recount stories of other women's breast cancer, forgetting that it can be immensely distressing to keep hearing tales about those who died from it.

I've sat through dinner parties where that became so painful to endure. You're trying to hold it together and not make it all about your illness for a change, when suddenly someone starts saying how awful it was for their friend – complete with all the gory details. And then comes the punchline that they died. If you've lost someone to breast cancer, hold back on telling us about it, because we need success stories to pull us through. We have enough doubts and fears of our own, without you adding to them. If your story doesn't have a happy ending, it's not one we want to hear.

What not to say

Here are just a few of the eye-wateringly insensitive things that have been said to other breast cancer patients. Avoid them at all costs. They'll go down like a lead balloon.

- You've got the good kind of cancer.

- Think of all the weight you'll lose.

- It's only hair – don't worry, it will grow back.

- If you wear a wig, it'll make you look like you don't have cancer.

- They've cut it out now, so you don't have to worry about it.

- You don't look sick.

- Everything happens for a reason.

- What did you do that made you get cancer?

- Maybe God is calling you home.

- Your cancer really depresses me.

- My aunt died of your cancer, but she had two good years.

The principles of what to say and what not to say aren't difficult. It just takes a little sensitivity and an ability to put yourself in someone else's shoes. If you don't know what to say, just listen and empathize. Make an effort to understand how we're feeling, rather than assuming you know. Don't make your beliefs more important than ours. Believe in us. We're stronger than you know. We've put that to the test.

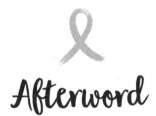

Afterword

'Above all, be the heroine of your life, not the victim.'

Nora Ephron

Sometimes it can be hard for me to believe I'm on the other side of this now. Breast cancer has consumed me for so many years that there are moments when I still struggle to believe that my life doesn't have to be about it anymore. Yet there are so many days now that pass without ever thinking of it, with so many more to come. The joy of forgetting is in letting go of the experience and living the lessons.

Part of the ability to let it go is the acceptance that it's served its purpose. While writing *Stronger Than Before*, I was graced with one of those moments we always wish we could have. Suddenly, I not only understood the purpose of my illness, but I felt the perfection of it too. I got it. I could see and feel the value of the changes that it had brought to my life. Not in a Pollyanna kind of way, just putting a positive spin on it, but in a genuine, heartfelt acceptance that it had a powerful role to play in my life – and one that was needed.

Would I consciously have chosen this path? Not for a New York minute. But I see what has changed within me and in the way I live my life, and ultimately it has all been worth it. I'm not the same woman who walked into the storm. And that's a very good thing.

Breast cancer is a wrecking ball. It will knock your house down to the foundations, and maybe even dig those out for good measure. But what grows back in its place can be so much more beautiful. Don't miss this opportunity. Be open to its dark gifts. A new strength, a new life and a new purpose await you.

References

Chapter 1: The Gathering Storm

1. www.nejm.org/doi/full/10.1056/NEJMp1401875
2. www.bmj.com/content/348/bmj.g366
3. https://breast-cancer-research.biomedcentral.com /articles/10.1186/s13058-015-0605-0
4. www.ncbi.nlm.nih.gov/pubmed/15197090
5. www.mbcn.org/incidence-and-incidence-rates
6. www.wsj.com/articles/some-cancer-experts-see-overdiagnosis-and-question-emphasis-on-early-detection-1410724838
7. *Tripping Over the Truth*, Travis Christofferson, foreword by Dominic D'Agostino, xii
8. www.cancerresearchuk.org/about-cancer/causes-of-cancer /inherited-cancer-genes-and-increased-cancer-risk/inherited-genes-and-cancer-types#inherited_genes1
9. www.nytimes.com/2016/05/15/magazine/warburg-effect-an-old-idea-revived-starve-cancer-to-death.html
10. Ibid.

Chapter 2: The Eye of the Storm

1. www.cancer.gov/about-cancer/causes-prevention/genetics/brca-fact-sheet

2. www.thelancet.com/journals/lanonc/article/PIIS1470-2045(17)30891-4/abstract

3. jamanetwork.com/journals/jama/fullarticle/1900512

4. www.sciencedaily.com/releases/2016/11/161123124443.htm

5. http://stm.sciencemag.org/content/9/397/eaan0026

6. www.ncbi.nlm.nih.gov/pubmed/15630849

7. www.sciencedaily.com/releases/2014/04/140406214413.htm

8. http://medicalphysicsweb.org/cws/article/research/53113

9. www.breastcancer.org/research-news/effect-of-radiation-on-reconstruction-results

10. http://newsroom.ucla.edu/releases/radiation-treatments-generate-229002

11. http://ascopubs.org/doi/abs/10.1200/JCO.1993.11.3.485

12. www.thelancet.com/journals/lanonc/article/PIIS1470-2045(14)71171-4/abstract

13. www.ncbi.nlm.nih.gov/pmc/articles/PMC2690973

14. www.ncbi.nlm.nih.gov/pubmed/21354370

15. www.bmj.com/content/359/bmj.j4530

16. www.ncbi.nlm.nih.gov/pubmed/11347286

17. www.ncbi.nlm.nih.gov/pubmed/18025276

18. http://mct.aacrjournals.org/content/10/7/1161.full

19. www.ncbi.nlm.nih.gov/pubmed/12181239

20. www.ncbi.nlm.nih.gov/pubmed/16338853

21. www.ncbi.nlm.nih.gov/pmc/articles/PMC3510426

22. www.ncbi.nlm.nih.gov/pmc/articles/PMC3673985

23. www.cancer.gov/about-cancer/treatment/cam/patient/vitamin-c-pdq#link/_9

24. www.ncbi.nlm.nih.gov/pubmed/17502596

25. www.ncbi.nlm.nih.gov/pubmed/15061657

26. https://gerson.org/gerpress/the-gerson-therapy

27. www.ncbi.nlm.nih.gov/pubmed/26934299

28. www.ncbi.nlm.nih.gov/pubmed/29116467

29. www.ncbi.nlm.nih.gov/pubmed/18712169
30. www.ncbi.nlm.nih.gov/pubmed/15623462

Chapter 3: No Mud, No Lotus

1. http://actualisedaily.com/wellbeing/the-cancer-personality

Chapter 4: Embodiment

1. www.physiology.org/doi/full/10.1152/ajpgi.1999.277.5.g922
2. www.ncbi.nlm.nih.gov/pubmed/8230262
3. http://cancerres.aacrjournals.org/content/canres/49/16/4373.full.pdf
4. www.ncbi.nlm.nih.gov/pmc/articles/PMC3195546/
5. www.ewg.org/foodnews/dirty_dozen_list.php#.WibJM7acaqA
6. www.ewg.org/foodnews/clean_fifteen_list.php#.WibJUbacaqA
7. www.ncbi.nlm.nih.gov/pubmed/12529346
8. https://articles.mercola.com/sites/articles/archive/2013/06/30/dagostino-cancer-research.aspx
9. www.ncbi.nlm.nih.gov/pubmed/27032109
10. www.ncbi.nlm.nih.gov/pubmed/28778338
11. www.aicr.org/continuous-update-project/reports/breast-cancer-report-2017.pdf
12. www.ncbi.nlm.nih.gov/pubmed/23638734
13. www.ncbi.nlm.nih.gov/pubmed/29152146
14. www.ncbi.nlm.nih.gov/pmc/articles/PMC3243677
15. https://silentspring.org/press-releases/scientists-identify-highest-priority-toxic-chemicals-target-breast-cancer-prevention
16. www.ncbi.nlm.nih.gov/pmc/articles/PMC3682794
17. www.ewg.org/skindeep/#.WnHDobacaqA
18. www.cmaj.ca/content/189/7/E268
19. www.ncbi.nlm.nih.gov/pubmed/24559833

Chapter 5: Emotional Ease

1. www.ncbi.nlm.nih.gov/pubmed/17903349
2. www.ncbi.nlm.nih.gov/pubmed/18394317
3. www.sciencedirect.com/science/article/pii/S1876382014003072
4. www.ajpmonline.org/article/S0749-3797(98)00017-8/abstract
5. www.cdc.gov/violenceprevention/acestudy/about.html

Chapter 7: Soulfulness

1. www.iwrotethisforyou.me/2012/06/grand-distraction.html

Chapter 8: Lotus in Bloom

1. www.breastcancercare.org.uk/about-us/media/press-releases/1-in-4-women-find-end-treatment-hardest-part-breast-cancer

Acknowledgements

The first glimmer of possibility that I could do this differently came through reading **Janet Edwards'** book, *Choosing to Heal: Surviving the Breast Cancer System*. It gave me hope to read about a real-life experience of overcoming breast cancer outside standard treatment in the UK and believe it could be possible for me. I have **David Cripps** to thank for recommending Janet's book and starting me on the path that became *Stronger Than Before*.

Then **Kris Carr** became my spirit animal for cancer nutrition, and I began to rely on my coaching and counselling training and all the teachings that had inspired me throughout my life to see me through. **Louise Hay** was my first port of call. I'd read her first book when it was still a small pamphlet, and without her trailblazing wisdom I would not have developed my own approach to healing breast cancer.

I called on everything I'd ever learned from the spiritual psychology of *A Course In Miracles*, my training as an interfaith minister and spiritual teachers like

Marianne Williamson and **Sanaya Roman**. Suddenly I became enormously grateful for the course junkie tendencies that had led me to study with **Miranda Macpherson, Robert Holden, Caroline Myss, Ian White, Baeth Davis, Marilyn Alauria, Robbi Zeck, Liesel Rigsby** and so many others. This book has been a lifetime in the making. Everything has been grist for the mill.

I was blessed with two amazing surgeons – **Mr Brendan Smith** in Reading for my cancer surgeries and **Mr Titus Adams** in Oxford for my reconstruction. Mr Smith, I will always be grateful that you tried to conserve my breast, even though you thought it probably wouldn't work. Mr Adams, you're a master. Your work is beautiful and I cannot tell you how much I appreciate that you took on the reduction at the same time as the reconstruction, saving me from yet another surgery. You have an incredible team too. The **BRA Group** is a superb resource for reconstruction patients, **Claire Griggs** is hands down the best breast cancer nurse I have ever met, and the nurses who looked after me during my week-long stay at the John Radcliffe were so thoughtful and caring.

Two wonderful women who are integrative doctors gave me the support and advice that I so desperately needed to carve my own path. **Dr Rosy Daniel** in Bath guided me on treatments beyond standard care and **Dr Nicola Hembry** in Bristol advised me on taking the Greece Test and working with its results. With their help, I could pursue evidence-based options and navigate my way through a constantly changing sea of information without drowning in it.

My friends are the ones who really got me through. They drove me to hospital appointments, made me laugh, cried with me, brought me food, fed the cat, celebrated the good times with me and did a thousand other little things that had a huge impact on how I coped and how I healed. They are legion, and so they shall have to remain nameless for fear of leaving someone out. They have my heart and a gratitude that will never die. In Henley, London, abroad and online, you showed how much you care and you all made a difference in your own way. I'm so lucky to have you in my life.

And then came **Hay House**. When my reconstruction was unexpectedly postponed, I decided to go to their Writer's Workshop, to make the best of the situation and do something I couldn't have done if the operation had gone ahead. From that weekend sprang the book, and my proposal won the competition and a contract. I can't thank **Michelle Pilley, Amy Kiberd, Jo Burgess, Julie Oughton and the rest of the team** enough for supporting *Stronger Than Before* from its earliest beginnings.

I cannot close without acknowledging a presence that has been with me every step of the way. From suffering the indignity of cuddles to help me recover, to camping out on my keyboard whenever he thought I needed a break, a little fat grumpy cat was my constant companion on the journey. Devastatingly, he lost his life as I put the finishing touches to these words. He was a holy terror – and Facebook-famous for it – but the sight of his furry face never failed to put a smile on mine. **Fatty**, this one's for you.

ABOUT THE AUTHOR

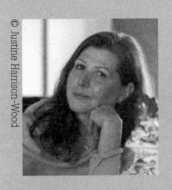

© Justine Harrison-Wood

Alison Porter is a journalist, coach, spiritual counsellor and interfaith minister. After an eclectic career that included film production, publishing and a high-profile corporate life heading up PR divisions for the Channel Tunnel and sale of the Millennium Dome – all while pursuing her interests in spiritual psychology – Alison's journey with breast cancer began in early 2015. She is now celebrating a cancer-free life after taking an unconventional approach to treatment.

Originally from Australia and now based in the UK, Alison utilized a lifetime's learning in spiritual and self-help techniques to help her overcome her illness, and to create the roadmap for healing that is *Stronger Than Before*.

Her work is now focused on supporting women with breast cancer – coaching them through all stages of their illness, helping them to make the choices that are right for them and empowering them through self-care. She sees breast cancer as a transformational process that can catalyse enormous post-traumatic growth – bringing the potential for a life of far greater meaning, joy and purpose than ever before.

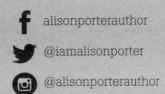

f alisonporterauthor

𝕏 @iamalisonporter

◎ @alisonporterauthor

www.alisonporter.co.uk

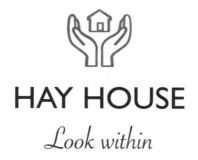

HAY HOUSE
Look within

Join the conversation about latest products, events, exclusive offers and more.

 f Hay House UK

 🐦 @HayHouseUK

 📷 @hayhouseuk

💜 healyourlife.com

We'd love to hear from you!